40 DAYS TO FREEDOM

"I'd been struggling for the last few years to figure out how to balance exercise and diet and in 5 weeks I've lost just over 9lbs.

It's been fabulous!

My body's gone through a lot of changes. I'm seeing my abs again for the first time in years!"

~ Stephanie S.

"When I picked up '40 Days to Freedom' it was the title that drew me in. I was hoping it was going to reignite something in me even though I felt my relationship with eating was something I had conquered.

I am still early on in my 40 day journey but am already hooked by the way I am challenged to participate from day one to rediscover my truest beliefs and values, to start from my unique place.

"Freedom to one person may be like prison to another..."
I love the way Ben and Suzanne have made each chapter into a manageable day of reading and reflecting. Though I have no idea what the results will be for me personally I already know it will be life changing!"

~ Meaghan M.

"So I'm halfway through and I would like to give myself a shout out. I went to TWO kid birthday parties and did not eat cake at either one. For me, this is huge!!! Slowly making changes and feeling it."

~ Rebecca S.

"40 Days To Freedom" not only educates the reader about why people have particular cravings, Ben and Suzanne provide a clear-cut plan on what to do about those cravings.

They go beyond the physical aspects of sugar addiction and illustrate perhaps the biggest factor at play, which is the psychological element.

I found the written exercises in the book to be a valuable tool as they really make you focus and reflect on what your individual value, belief, and goal systems are and get down to the rawness of what makes you, you."

~ Mike R.

"It was a pleasure working with Ben and Suzanne. I'm so happy with the results I've received and everything that I've learned to maintain my good health.

I can't begin to explain in words how wonderful it's been to work through these issues and feel like myself again when I had so much despair before."

~ Carrie C.

"This book is an incredible tool that guides the way, simply and clearly to uncovering controlling programming, releasing the negative patterns that are holding you back and then creating empowering new ones to give you power and drive to achieve your individual goals...and FREEDOM!

'40 Days to Freedom' is a very easy read that gives so many insights and action steps for you to follow. As long as you take action, you are guaranteed to see a transformation."

~ Veronica B.

"It was great, I didn't expect to get the results that I got. In less than 40 days I lost 2% body fat and 6.3 inches in different places from my body. I could tell it was working when a pair of jeans I could barely fit into before starting the program were fitting loosely in only 2 weeks' time!

I kinda knew what we were doing but it seemed unreal until the changes started happening...then it suddenly felt very real!

What's amazing is that in 6 months I lost a whopping 33.5 inches and 8.6% body fat!

Thank you very much!"

~ Dipika K.

"I started working with Ben and Suzanne after suffering a rather extreme case of adrenal fatigue while tackling a graduate program and working full time.

I felt so horrible I was inclined to go towards more extreme measures.

After a long review of my situation, Ben and Suzanne recommended trying a more balanced approach.

They gave me supplement recommendations that were far more affordable than most and within two to three days of taking them, I was already feeling better.

Fortunately Ben & Suzanne have a very holistic view of health and can make easy and affordable tweaks that help me regain balance and either feel a lot better or perform a lot better."

~ Ravi C.

40 DAYS to FREEDOM

Shed the Shackles of
Food Craving, Diet Cycling
& Body Shaming

BEN PATWA
SUZANNE CATHERINE

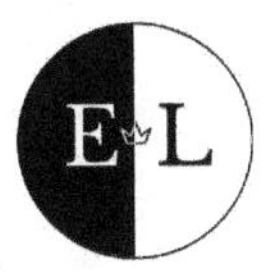

40 DAYS to FREEDOM

Shed the Shackles of Food Craving, Diet Cycling & Body Shaming

Disclaimer: Understand that the information contained in this book is opinion, and should be used for personal educational purposes only. You are responsible for your own behavior, and this book is not to be considered medical, legal, or personal advice. Nor is this book to be understood as putting forth any cure for any type of acute or chronic psychological or physiological illness. Please check with your physician before making any changes recommended in this book.

Published by Experts Legacy Publishing.
www.ExpertsLegacyPublishing.com

Cover Art: M Jordan Raspatie.
Back Cover Photo: Sarah Orbanic.

ISBN: 0692692835
ISBN-13: 978-0692692837

Dedication

This book is dedicated to our parents Amir & Rita and David & Catherine for instilling in us the drive to be the best we can be in service to others.

Thank you to our children Vivian & Dash for their support, patience and comic relief throughout this writing endeavor.

Special thanks to Coach Doe Williams, Mrs. Betty Bridge and all of those who've supported us in becoming the people we are today.

May this book be a big part of our legacy and serve as inspiration for many others to leave their own.

Ben & Suzanne

Claim your support materials here.

It has been a long-held goal of ours to create a paradigm shift in the way that the world views and approaches health.

Our mission is to empower adults as well as children to find *their* unique definitions of freedom, to live by their own guidelines and to follow their path despite any negative influence from the media, society or people around them.

We have created a number of supporting resources that accompany the processes you'll experience in this book, including:

- Video trainings
- Guided audios
- Downloadable worksheets
- Recipes & guides

These are included as our gift to help you create the most effective and lasting change possible.

40DaysToFreedom.com/reso
urces

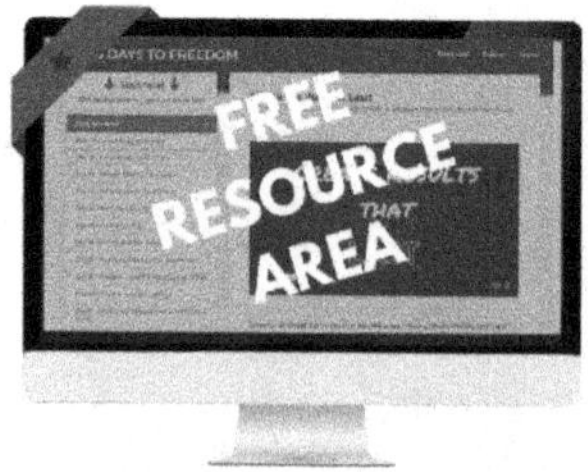

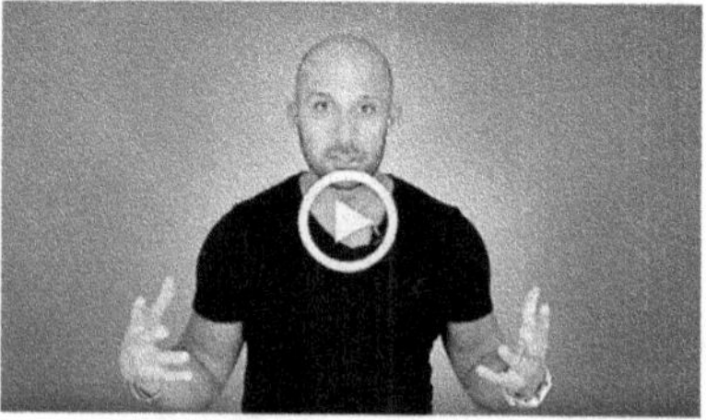

Table Of Contents

The best time to plant a tree was 20 years ago; the second best time is now.

~ Chinese Proverb

Authors' Preface

Ben:

This book is the product of a journey that started far before my interest in health and fitness began. Back when it was one thing, the *only* thing...the rest is just details kinda thing. Basketball.

I look up and see the sweaty giant approaching, his steps falling into slow motion as the sound of the crowd fades and the images in my periphery begin to blur. I am alone as the sole guardian of the basket, as a much larger man charges toward me. I am twelve. My awareness is soon limited to him, the ball, and remembering what I was taught to do in that situation....take a charge.

Taking a charge means standing absolutely still and vulnerable in front of the opponent and remaining still until he hits me, earning a foul.
Well, he hit me...HARD.

What happened next would shape my character and influence the rest of my life.

After bulldozing over me and I think, making the basket (I was a little dazed on the ground to know for sure), I heard the whistle blow. The referee had called "charge", an offensive foul. Soon my opponent was being screamed at by his head coach, pointing out how a young, little boy like me had out-witted him, playing the game better and winning the respect and admiration of the rest of the team.

As I got up I felt myself stand taller and feel more certain about being willing to do what's necessary, even if I was scared!

This incident or Significant Emotional Event (S.E.E.), unbeknownst to me at the time, would ultimately be a catalyst to committing to live in line with the values I care about - responsibility, honor and courage – no matter what.

At the age of 18, I had another S.E.E. that would catapult me into the world of holistic health studies, nutrition and performance psychology...one that ultimately led to writing this book with my partner Suzanne Catherine.

Shortly after reaching the highest point of my basketball career, winning Gold in a championship against 22 teams from around the world, I was admitted to the hospital with failure of 2 major organs!

This near-death experience was analogous to a heart attack at 50. It woke me up and rattled me to the core. I now understood how fragile life can be, and from that moment, I would stand for nothing short of excellence in my life. Furthermore, I would commit to helping to foster excellence in others, whether in health, relationships, business, or personal growth. This book is in part a manifestation of that commitment.

We wrote '40 Days to Freedom' as a way to open the reader's mind to the unconscious actions and reactions that are constantly going on inside of us. How we interpret the outcome affects how we feel, then serves to create beliefs that solidify our values and in turn, influences our behavior.

This book will take you on your own journey, exploring how certain beliefs or patterns got created for you, and empowering you with tools, tips and processes to help you break free from the shackles that have encumbered you. We wish you well!

Suzanne:

When I was sixteen, I was invited to compete in a Junior Olympic girls' volleyball national qualifying meet. I had been playing club volleyball all over the state during the summer before my Junior year of high school, and had been selected to travel to a neighboring state to compete for a spot on the U.S. Junior Olympic Team.

My ass was kicked in the first round and I was quickly eliminated.

Nevertheless, I continued to excel at the sport and finished my Junior year season strongly, already being scouted for college volleyball scholarships.

Then, in early summer before my Senior year, I made a decision that would alter my course dramatically. All of the hours of practice, winning games and early accolades were tossed aside in pursuit of thinner thighs. I chose an eating disorder instead.

Over the course of two months my athletic frame was reduced by 20 pounds. At last, the extraordinarily muscular thighs that marred my body image could squeeze into a size 2. I had made it over to the 'feminine' side.

Until that summer, for as long as I could remember, I hated my legs. They weren't like the other girls'. My friends had lovely, lean ballerina legs that looked pretty under skirts. Mine took interesting, globular forms. Striations appeared with the slightest tension. My quads spilled over my knees. I felt the strength of my legs and knew their benefits, however I struggled with wanting to feel more feminine, and coveted a girlish frame.

Through my extreme dieting, as well as losing any hint of breasts I had, I lost my period, too. Ironically, my quest for smaller, more 'feminine' thighs snuffed out the very essence of femininity I already possessed.

Although my anorexia/bulimia was short-lived, I remained generally uninformed on the topic of nutrition through my 20's, occasionally dabbling with the latest fad diet or whatever my closest circle of friends were eating, out of convenience or economics.

With the beginning of my 30's came young motherhood. I now had two children, a flailing marriage and a physique that reflected my perpetually stressed state. I was 40 pounds overweight, overwrought and undernourished – physically, emotionally and spiritually. My low self-esteem and resulting limiting beliefs about who I could be and what was possible in my situation would paralyze me for years.

Finally, the pain and fear of remaining the same outweighed the fear of making a change. Initially, it was the love I had for my children that sparked my desire. They were getting older and their awareness was expanding...I refused to be responsible for their witnessing the pain, isolation and desperation their mother endured as the result of her self-neglect. I wanted them to know nothing of opportunities missed as a result of my lack of confidence.

I wanted them to have the opportunity to model a mother who loved herself so much that she could stand in all of her vulnerability, rawness, pain and weakness and despite it all, have the courage, grit and stamina to press confidently toward her dreams.

Making changes to my home environment and with newfound energy flowing, I began my quest for knowledge in nutrition and fitness. Years of experience in my nursing career had firmly implanted the importance of good health and its benefits – as well as the awareness of the dire consequences for those who neglected it. I had seen awful things, and I didn't want them to happen to me.

I read countless books and had countless conversations. I gleaned wisdom from my own experimentation. The pounds melted away as I implemented what I learned, and let go of the weight of emotional baggage. My sense of well-being and confidence soared, as did my career, wealth and relationships. I met my greatest Love and co-author of this book, Ben Patwa.

Together, guided by his coaching brilliance and nutrition/exercise expertise, my indomitable will, and our studies in Neuro-Linguistic Programming (NLP), I continued my physical and emotional evolution and fulfilled a once-frightening goal to compete in an international fitness competition...at the age of 40.

In addition to the obvious dedication to my fitness and nutrition regime that was required, by deleting destructive mental patterns and installing new beliefs about myself, I earned second place and took home two trophies. If the 16 year-old version of me could see into her future, she'd have been amused to see those muscular thighs in a new (fluorescent!) light.

I am so grateful to have earned this platform as fitness model to inspire and empower others to become the best version of themselves! To that end, it is an honor to have my voice included in the pages of this powerfully transformative book. Enjoy your journey to FREEDOM!

Introduction

As a conscious health consumer, does the vast amount of information available online, in bookstores, from health professionals and peers only leave you feeling overwhelmed and unsure of whom to trust, and what to implement?

Do you encounter conflicting and confusing information seemingly at every turn, leaving you with more questions than answers?

Have you come to realize that having the best intentions or strong "willpower" to gain control over your eating habits isn't enough to thrust you out of an addictive cycle?

Perhaps you've perceived to have some success with a particular diet, only to find yourself rebound back to the same or worse condition over time - now weighted with the compounded effects of exasperation, desperation and despair guiding your choices.

You may be a new recipient of a concerning medical diagnosis, a parent seeking healthful alternatives to the standard school lunch fare or convenience dinner foods, or an athlete seeking a competitive advantage... and you are all left with the same question: How do I break free from the rut or routine where I seem to be trapped?

As you sift through mountains of literature on the latest fad diet or scientific study, as you consider and sometimes succumb to gimmicky "shortcuts" and home machines that are "guaranteed" to deliver gleaming health - you grow sicker, fatter and more frustrated.

There is no diet, no exclusive or restrictive pattern that ever works for humans long-term. It is hardwired into our being to break out of these patterns. That is why most attempts for us to simply "willpower our way there" end in misery, disappointment and even do damage to our metabolisms.

There is not one definition of freedom that is the right definition for everyone. We are all unique biochemical beings, with distinct physical and emotional differences. We cannot expect to experience the same results of another's experimentation toward better health, nor can we rely on lab research that does not translate into the human experience, and its diverse population.

Our unique expression of humanness and our perception of well-being is a complex and savory stew of our internal representations of what it means to be healthy, as well as distinctly measurable external variables. We have different ancestries, different metabolic types, different health histories and different health goals.
So what can be taught in one book that could serve the health of the masses? Keep reading, you'll soon know.

40 DAYS to FREEDOM leads the reader through an expertly guided transformational process to break the cycle of food craving, diet cycling & body shaming, once and for all.

Using Neuro-Linguistic Programming (NLP), we will teach you how to overcome compulsions and bad habits, and to release limiting beliefs and emotional connections to food.

By implementing the steps found in this book you will re-program the way you think and feel about your body and install positive and supportive habits that keep you accountable and progressing toward your goals.

With your newfound knowledge and motivation you will become equipped and empowered to create lasting results.

We have created many resources to help you through key concepts of this book in audio, visual and experiential formats.

Visit **http://40DaysToFreedom.com/resources** to download what you need, watch instructional videos and hear the guided success audios to help you on your journey.

This book is for people who are fed up with feeling tired, unmotivated, foggy and frazzled. It is for the person who wants to feel energized, sexy, fit of body and clear of mind. It is for anyone who is ready to be free to live a life realizing their greatest potential, unencumbered by disease. It is for the person who has "tried everything", and is desperate to find the right path.

Why place your trust in us to lead you toward that path? We have collectively spent 30+ years helping others transform their lives through the practices of Nursing, Functional Diagnostic Nutrition, Physiotherapy, Corrective Exercise Therapy, NLP, Hypnotherapy, Mental & Emotional Release Therapy and Behavioral Change Therapy.

We have created thousands of personalized nutrition and fitness programs including metabolic typing and natural hormone balancing, helping clients to lose weight, build lean muscle, increase libido and boost energy and performance.

Women have reported more regular menstrual cycles, mood stability, and significantly diminished or even complete cessation in menopausal symptoms.

Members of corporations have reported benefiting from increased productivity and satisfaction along with better team cohesion and retention from our comprehensive and individualized wellness programs.

Ben successfully built his holistic practice and expert reputation both hands-on in his privately owned London clinic and with clients spanning the globe.

He became a lifetime student of holistic health studies following his near-death experience when he suffered multiple organ failure at the young age of eighteen.

His resulting resolve to uncover how his body works and his commitment to helping others has fueled his passion for excellence in his field.

He is popularly known as **"The guy you go to when nothing else has worked"**.

Suzanne has nearly two decades of healthcare experience in the nursing profession, the majority of which has been spent in Intensive Care Units in some of the top-ranked hospitals in North America.

Troubled by the common diagnoses she saw in so many patients - Coronary Artery Disease, Peripheral Vascular Disease, Stroke, Cardiac Arrest, Obesity, Diabetes Type 2 - and learning that so many of them are preventable with education, availability of resources, a shift in lifestyle and the desire to live well, she transitioned into private nursing to have a greater impact on her patients through holistic education and healing.

She has personally run the gamut of physical shapes and sizes, from athletic to anorexic to significantly overweight... to successful competitive fitness model.

She has experienced living with borderline obesity, shackled to sugar addiction and the effects of hormonal imbalance following pregnancies, before her studies and the influence of Ben taught her how to navigate the process to freedom so many of our readers are desperate to achieve.

Using the guidelines we describe in this book, Suzanne has been able to maintain her exceptional level of fitness and model physique for years.

She often says, ***"Once I knew better, I couldn't forget. This knowledge changed the way I think about food and exercise, and most important, the way I view myself. I simply could not go back to being the person I used to be."***

She does not stand alone in her success.

Here is what some of Suzanne's and Ben's clients are saying:

"I'd been struggling for the last few years to figure out how to balance exercise and diet and in only 5 weeks I've lost just over 9lbs and it's been fabulous! My body's gone through a lot of changes. I'm seeing my abs again for the first time in years!"

~ *Stephanie S.*

"I was struggling with how I looked and felt. I was desperate to lose weight. I was eating what I thought was healthy and visiting the gym regularly but wasn't getting results. I was tested to see what my Metabolic Type was and I soon discovered I was eating all the wrong foods.

My goal was to feel happy and comfortable in my bikini on my holiday.

It worked, it was amazing!

In 16 weeks I dropped 4 dress sizes, my energy levels improved dramatically and I felt amazing. This is a way of life, no quick fixes. It's not a diet, it's a lifestyle.

Once you understand how it works it's incredibly easy to maintain."

.

~ *Elizabeth W.*

"I was having some issues with lack of energy and a general feeling of malaise throughout the day. I was relying heavily on caffeine and other stimulants to power me through my weightlifting and running sessions.

I was referred to Ben and Suzanne to help me look for the underlying cause of my problems.

They "held my hand" as they broke all the scientific jargon down into layman's terms so that I could see just what was going on.

I followed their plan, took the recommended supplements and started to get back to normal energy levels within a few weeks!

I would highly recommend trusting in the advice of Ben and Suzanne to anyone who is looking to feel better, get stronger, more fit and stabilize their energy levels as well as increase their sense of well-being."

~ Mike R.

"It was a pleasure working with Ben and Suzanne. I'm so happy with the results I've received and everything that I've learned to maintain my good health.

I can't begin to explain in words how wonderful it's been to work through these issues and feel like myself again when I had so much despair before."

~ Carrie C.

"It was great, I didn't expect to get the results that I got. In less than 40 days I lost 2% body fat and 6.3 inches in different places from my body. I could tell it was working when a pair of jeans I could barely fit into before starting the program were fitting loosely in only 2 weeks' time!

I kinda knew what we were doing but it seemed unreal until the changes started happening...then it suddenly felt very real!

What's amazing is that in 6 months I lost a whopping 33.5 inches and 8.6% body fat!

Thank you very much!"

~ Dipika K.

"I started working with Ben and Suzanne after suffering a rather extreme case of adrenal fatigue while tackling a graduate program and working full time.

I felt so horrible I was inclined to go towards more extreme measures.

After a long review of my situation, Ben and Suzanne recommended trying a more balanced approach.

They gave me supplement recommendations that were far more affordable than most and within two to three days of taking them, I was already feeling better.

Fortunately Ben & Suzanne have a very holistic view of health and can make easy and affordable tweaks that help me regain balance and either feel a lot better or perform a lot better."

~ Ravi C.

Ben and Suzanne have helped people of all ages and all walks of life to achieve their goals including postpartum mothers, brides-to-be, film and television celebrities, government officials, fitness competitors and professional athletes. Collectively their clients have lost countless pounds, have recovered from devastating illness and injury, and have built the strength and stamina to powerfully create the lives of their dreams.

So, what's in this for you? We **boldly** promise that when you implement what we outline in this book, you will not only get rid of food addictions and finally let go of "dieting", you will become equipped and empowered to make lasting change.

You WILL feel better, guaranteed.

Our methods are so effective because they blend ancient wisdom and tried-and-true, old-fashioned clean eating with human psychology, Neuro-linguistic programming (NLP) and decades of clinical experience in behavior change. There is no gimmick, no cookie-cutter plan, no pill or miracle machine. If you are ready to receive this information and implement it, if you are truly ready to commit to change, *do not live another day without this book*.

It will change your life for the better.

We promise.

**Freedom is not given
to us by anyone;
we have to
cultivate it ourselves.
It is a daily practice.**

~ Thich Nhat Hanh

Day 40

Countdown To Freedom

This marks your first day on your path to freedom. Simply by picking up this book you have taken a vital action step toward achieving freedom. How you continue is up to *you*.

We want to congratulate you for your commitment to continuing! Yes, by simply reading this line you have chosen to read on from the last paragraph, and you're still moving forward. This is congruent with the habits that will bring you success on this endeavor!

Often it is the ordinary things, done consistently over time, that create extraordinary results.

We have started with day 40 because this is a count*down*. Psychologically our minds like shrinking numbers. We like simplicity and we like to feel closer to rather than farther from something we want.

Each word you consume, each page you digest, each chapter you absorb will bring you closer and closer to freedom.

It will sneak up on you.

You may not realize all of the changes that have happened to you as you progress through the unique structure of this book.

You may wake up one day noticing you've changed, or someone you haven't seen in a while will bump into you and call out your huge transformation.

You might even shrug it off, because you focused on making small, incremental changes by continuing to read and follow the action steps and have made this such a way of life that you no longer remember what it used to be like to be the "old you" - trapped and chained to food addiction.

You may find it difficult to retrieve the feeling of what it was like to be in a perpetual cycle of dieting and shaming of your body, and other people's bodies.

Thankfully you will perhaps no longer feel the unhappiness you used to feel as a result, either.

What we share with you on the next page may be one of the most important concepts for your entire journey.

It's not your fault.

If you have surpassed the age of five you have likely already suffered a barrage of unhealthy influences in your lifetime. Uninformed caregivers, unscrupulous food companies and artful advertisers have crept into your subconscious mind, laying pathways to a prison where sugar has swallowed the key.

As a youngster, a tumble off the tricycle and a resulting skinned knee might have provoked a well-meaning mama to shower you with loving attention, including a sweet chocolate kiss among her own. A sugary remedy offered by a trusted hand, in an emotional moment, to ease the pain...and so the neuro-association with sugar satisfying pain had begun.

Candy as a reward for accomplishment as well as countless sweet celebrations, where happy decorated cakes sent waves of reinforcing neurotransmitters shouting, “YES! Sugar = Happy Times!” have left you feeling powerless against their advances in adulthood. Is there any wonder why so many of us turn to sugary foods to subconsciously recreate the happy feelings associated with these events when we feel we need a little uplifting?

It’s not your fault.

We create unsupportive beliefs and neuro-associations (mind-connections) as a result of **Significant Emotional Events (S.E.E.’s)**. Sometimes the belief is formed slowly over a number of experiences, or, if the event is intense and/or sudden enough it can be formed in an instant!

Can you think of any Significant Emotional Events that happened in your early life in the area of health and fitness?

Think between the ages of 0-7 and 7-14. These are two critical periods when we are imprinted by the people and situations around us. We also form our initial beliefs and values during this time although they may have evolved or shifted since then due to other events.

Consider any past relationships that had an impact on how you felt about the way you look or the way others look. Maybe you heard derogatory remarks about your body over and over until you started to own it.

Consider your past experiences with food.

What was the conversation like?
Was it one of scarcity or indulgence?
How do you believe this has this affected you?

With these programs or beliefs or negative feelings installed into your operating system, has your life since been a constant battle between will and wanting?

Even when you thought you were avoiding the obvious emotional triggers to your sugarcoated cravings, food companies have enrolled you in a cycle of addiction perpetuated by the inclusion of sugar in a staggering array of products lining the supermarket shelves today.

The addictive substance is now often found in bottled sauces and dressings, condiments, breads, canned soups, sports drinks, energy bars, and several processed and packaged convenience foods. Recently, our supermarket search for spaghetti sauce revealed just ONE sauce out of twenty-three options that did not contain added sugar!

So-called "diet" foods are often laced with manufactured, sweet-tasting chemicals that not only exacerbate certain medical conditions, but cause a different kind of chemical reaction in your brain that sabotages your intentions to cut sugar from your diet.

How could this be? Why can consuming low-calorie or no-calorie artificial sugar products actually cause you to gain *more* weight? Calories in, calories out, right?

Wrong.

In the next chapter we'll reveal interesting facts about your brain chemistry, the chemical reactions that occur that sabotage your best efforts to create your desired results, and why it has become easy to be slaves to sugar, grains and alcohol in the modern world.

It's not your fault, however it *is* your responsibility to learn how to navigate it.

Your Two Brains

It's true, you have two, and they talk to each other.

One is located quite obviously within your skull. The other? It's in your gut! It's called the Enteric Nervous System, comprised of approximately 100 million nerve cells lining your gastrointestinal tract.

This little 'brain in your belly' is mainly responsible for releasing enzymes that aid in digestion by breaking down foods, for controlling blood flow that helps with nutrient absorption, and for communicating with your other brain how it feels about the food it's been receiving.

Studies have shown that the gut brain cannot only communicate when you're full, it also judges when you've eaten something nutritious, and when to keep looking for food!

Did you know that when you eat certain foods, despite the quantity you've eaten, your gut may tell you it's unsatisfied and to eat *more*?! This little brain analyzes the food you eat and sends messages up to your big brain about what is there, or what's missing.

When you eat artificially sweetened food, for example, your gut brain gets very confused. In nature anything that is sweet has a fair amount of nutrition that comes along with it.

The problem is that over the industrial revolution food companies and scientists have extracted, dried, squeezed or manufactured sweet things with virtually no nutrition.

Artificial sweeteners are typically 100-600 times sweeter per ounce than sugar and often have zero calories - and zero nutrition.

When your gut senses this, it sends a message to your brain that it was tricked and to keep looking for nutrition (food). Often the response is overeating!

This is just one example of how man-made food, or playing with nature's chemistry, can cause serious issues. It's one of the reasons why we've seen a huge expansion of waistlines commensurate with the growth of diet foods and drinks available today. (Hopefully that is enough to have you put down the diet soda once and for all)!

Another bit of brain science that may be of interest to you when seeking to understand why you have cravings and food addictions is recognizing the role of neurotransmitters in your body.

Neurotransmitters are like little chemical text messages sent between your brain and the trillions of cells that make up the systems of your body. They let glands and organs know what to do when there is an imbalance, automatically controlling the functioning of things to keep everything working behind the scenes.

The three neurotransmitters of particular interest within the context of this book are serotonin, beta-endorphin, and dopamine.

When serotonin is at an optimal level, we generally feel a sense of well-being, peace and optimism. We are also more likely to exhibit greater self-control as we tend to be more thoughtful and focused with our responses to our environment.

When serotonin is below an optimal level, we can experience feelings of depression and can be rather scattered and disorganized.

We may be more likely to act impulsively to satisfy our hunger to create the uplifting feeling that indulgence in refined carbohydrates like sugar, grains and alcohol can bring - albeit only temporarily.

We *crave* these foods. Our brains know what to trigger in us to create the intense urge to eat foods that will boost those serotonin levels. The urge is so gripping that we often succumb to these cravings, feeling immediate gratification with the subsequent high.

Sugar in not unlike a drug. Several studies have revealed that it has the same affect on our brains that drugs like heroin and amphetamines do.

Like heroin and amphetamines, sugar can have a devastating boomerang effect when the high wears off, sending its abusers into yet another cycle of using and crashing. The resulting negative emotions and health consequences only serve to perpetuate the problem.

As if serotonin seeking weren't a significant contributor, the feel-good effects of the neurotransmitter beta-endorphin add to your selective food addiction with its delivery of a highly valued sense of wellbeing and self-esteem.

Some people even enjoy a sense of euphoria when the "endorphin rush" kicks in. It's the ultimate physical and emotional painkiller, and can be bought cheaply and easily by adults and children alike most anywhere in the world.

Add the seductive effects of dopamine to the mix of brain chemicals designed to elevate alertness and mood with food and you've got yourself three very powerful motivators to continue your destructive cycle of binging on sugar and refined carbs.

Willpower and intention are often crushed by the brain's overriding message to lift you out of the depths of a rebound from the last meal where you "used" these foods.

The struggle is real, and it takes more than strong determination to break free of this cycle. We know because we've done it, and have led many others to freedom. Please read on to learn how you can do it, too.

Day 39

Get Defined.

It's not enough to know *why* you have the cravings - this knowledge means little unless you know *what* to do about it.

In order to shed the shackles of sugar and the seemingly endless cycle of dieting, you must build an army of combating forces that move indomitably toward freedom. This army cannot be bought, borrowed, or begged into existence.

It takes awareness and thoughtful recruiting for a tactical team to accompany and support you on your journey, and this team can only be assembled by *you*.

There is no one who knows you better than you know yourself, wouldn't you agree?
For this reason, you must own the responsibility to recruit the thoughts that you'll be thinking, create the environment where you'll be dwelling, and identify the path you'll be taking, to get to freedom.

What has worked for one person may not work for you.
Decide now to reject the idea that your results must be measured against someone else's. Aside from our differences and biochemical individuality, we all have different definitions of freedom! **We can only measure against ourselves.**

The first thing to do is to define what freedom means to *you*.
Imagine yourself, free.

What does being free from your food addictions look like?
What types of foods would remain?
What are your non-negotiables? In other words, what food or drink are you *unwilling* to give up, period.

Maybe it's the nightly sip of red wine, or Saturday morning pancakes with the family. Be honest with yourself. What can you see yourself living without, and what would you like to keep?

Of course, keeping everything that you're currently eating is probably not going to render the result you desire. Consider carefully what foods you know are contributing to the problem, yet to feel deprived of them would likely take you off course with frequent binging.

The good news is that you can eat the foods you love and still find freedom from their current power over you. You simply need to learn how to fit them into a lifestyle that is congruent with your goals.

Knowing when to eat them, how to eat them, and what activities to add or stop around their consumption - will help you build your unique "freedom formula" to achieve your desired outcome.

Applying this knowledge will help you to feel equipped and empowered to take actions and create results that last regardless of any changes or challenges that come up in your life!

My Freedom Values

Values are the primary drivers behind our behaviors. In other words, what we deem to be important to us influences the way we conduct our lives.

Values guide our actions because values are above behavior in our "neurological levels".

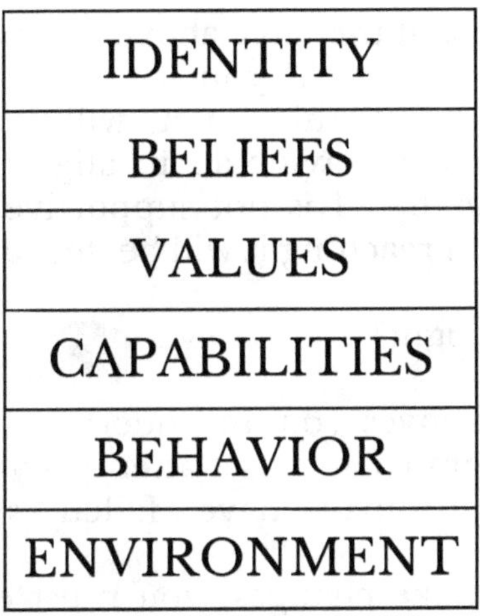

fig a) - System of Neurological Levels (top is highest)

This table can provide great insight because one can see clearly *what* influences *what* in the mind and body.
Identity is at the top and everything trickles down from there, influencing the level(s) below.

If your beliefs are the issue then you can imagine how that will affect what you value, what you feel that you are allowed or capable of doing, and even the environment that you will allow yourself to be in.

If you struggle with your behavior then look above to your values and below at your environment and you're sure to find some of the issues.

We aim to work with you throughout this book, and beyond if you feel that it is right, to help you to transform at every level. These shifts, like life, may come at you seemingly randomly and not in a linear fashion. This is so that your conscious mind and ego don't trick you into thinking or believing that you are on track and set you up to sabotage your success!

Simply looking at the table above we can see how that last statement works. If your mind or ego tricks you into believing something, you will set your values, capabilities and behavior all in alignment with that belief. If your belief is not supportive of your goal, your success in reaching it will be defeated.

Makes sense, right?

We hope this gives you an understanding as to why previous programs and past attempts you've made to make changes may have fallen short on the deliverables.
In order to make changes, you must examine these levels and make the necessary adjustments to each to reach your particular goals!

Let's talk about values.
Values are always correct. There is no true or false questionnaire or written test because there is no right or wrong when it comes to values. As we learned earlier, they are driven by our Identity and Beliefs and thus we make them correct by choosing our actions, shaping our environment and adapting our whole lives around them.

Your values may cause you to take massive, immediate action, like when standing up for something or protecting someone. They may also lead you to remain inactive, such as to allow someone else freedom or to give them what you perceive to be as giving respect.

What are your values? Consider what is important to you - so important that you will do just about anything for it.

Identify your Freedom Values:

On the next page you will find a table of common human values.

1. Read through these and with a pencil place a star next to the ones that resonate with you at first glance.

2. Write these out on a blank paper (or in a "Freedom Journal" that you create to go with this book).

3. Place them in order of your top 10.

4. Keep this safe as you will refer back to it later in the book and compare what has shifted and what has stayed the same.

Human Values

Abundance	**Freedom**	Prosperity
Accomplishment	Friendship	Purpose
Achievement	Fun	Recognition
Accountability	Gratitude	Regularity
Accuracy	Greatness	Relationships
Adventure	Growth	Reliability
Beauty	Happiness	Respect
Boldness	Hard work	Responsibility
Bravery	Harmony	Safety
Calm	Health	Satisfaction
Challenge	Honesty	Security
Change	Honor	Self-awareness
Choice	Improvement	Self-confidence
Collaboration	Independence	Self-giving
Commitment	Individuality	Self-reliance
Communication	Inner peace	Service
Community	Innovation	Simplicity
Comfort	Integrity	Skill
Compassion	Intuitiveness	Solving-Problems
Competence	Justice	Speed
Connection	Knowledge	Spontaneity
Cooperation	Leadership	Structure
Coordination	Learning	Success
Creativity	Love	Teamwork
Decisiveness	Loyalty	Timeliness
Discipline	Money	Tolerance
Diversity	Openness	Tradition
Effectiveness	Order	Transformation
Efficiency	Organization	Tranquility
Empowerment	Passion	Trust
Excellence	Peace	Truth
Exploration	Perfection	Unity
Fairness	Pleasure	Variety
Faith	Power	Wealth
Family	Preservation	Wisdom
Flexibility	Progress	

Now that you've identified your freedom values, it's important to find your **threshold** value(s).

Your threshold values are the "deal breakers". They are like the emergency eject button from a relationship, job or situation.

Think of a relationship. What if someone had their top 10 values present in it, and everything was great. The threshold value would be the one or number of things that would cause someone to bolt from that relationship even if all of the desired values were present.

Let's say communication, chemistry, quality time, and adventure were all present, yet maybe infidelity would cause someone to leave, no matter how great the situation is otherwise.

You may be thinking, "Of course, wouldn't everyone choose to leave if that happened?" and that wouldn't be true. We are all so unique that what we value and where we draw the lines of our boundaries is equally unique.
Think now about *your* threshold values. What would be so deeply violating for you that you would give up or leave a situation, even if it seemed to have everything else you wanted?

This is a powerful process to help you create more firm boundaries around behaviors, people, attitudes and circumstances that would violate what you deem as your core values.

This process can also show you why you may not have succeeded in achieving goals or targets in the past, especially if the perceived gain was trumped by what you saw as a threshold value toward staying the same and missing your target.

In the context of your health and relationship to food it may be that you would give up freedom instead of giving up indulgence, or the feeling of adventurous eating to achieve a fit and lean body.

Consider how this **conflict** of values may have sabotaged your success in the past, or influenced your choice to give up on completing a goal.

Use the same Human Values table to identify your threshold values, and while doing so be open to finding out a few more very important freedom values that you may have missed earlier.

Identify your Threshold Values:

1. Re-Read through the Human Values and look for any values that stand out as an "emergency eject button"!

2. Write these down too.

3. You will also refer back to these later and compare what has shifted and what has stayed the same.

To move a big rock, you must gain leverage.

Take a moment now to write down below how important it is for you to reclaim your freedom from food addictions. How liberating would it be to break free from society's definition of beauty, and gain control over your eating so you never need to diet again.

This process will serve as a huge lever to "move mountains" that may have blocked your path for years.

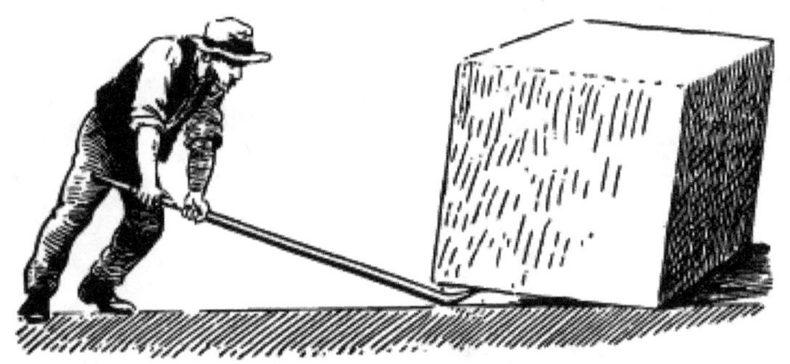

Day 38

Freedom Fingerprint

Your definition of freedom is so unique that it is analogous to a fingerprint and completely incomparable to someone else's.

Freedom to one person may be like prison to another, so for *YOU* to be successful it's important to know what your desired outcome (destination) will be, BEFORE you embark on the journey.

Imagine you've jumped into your car and have started driving with the idea that you'll use the GPS to help you get where you want to go.

What if you forgot to enter the *destination* of where you wanted to go? Would you still expect to get there? You'd essentially be driving blindly, right? Now imagine that your friend borrowed your car and the GPS was still programmed with their last destination. You certainly wouldn't get where *you* want to go and may end up somewhere entirely off course, and wrong for you.

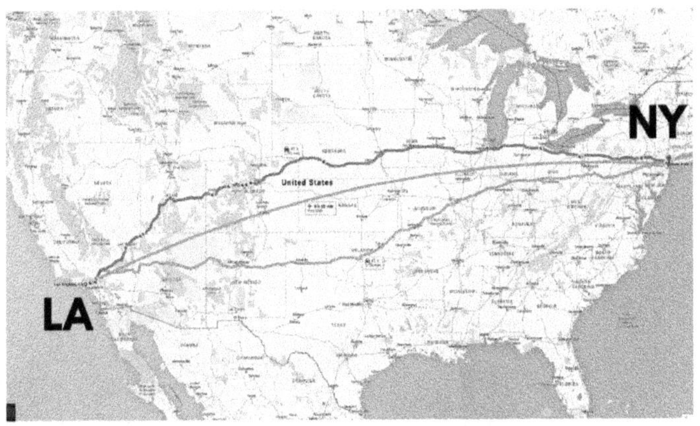

As much of an exaggerated example this is, it happens far too often when people take action without a plan. Many times people want to follow a path that worked for someone else.

The result could be disappointing, demotivating and even damaging as body shaming and negative associations with failed attempts are imprinted.

What's *Your* Success GPS?

Before you embark on your journey to freedom, you need to identify your starting point as well as your end point. The previous chapters will have hopefully helped to clarify these for you.

In addition to these points, you'll want to clearly outline all the possible paths to get there, otherwise you may find yourself on a path that you neither intended nor enjoy.

Next, you'll want to identify any obstacles or potential distractions that may take you off course. Be sure to factor in time for refilling gas and pee breaks! :)

Ask yourself these questions:

What are you going to do to get there?

What are you willing to do/not do?

Will you move methodically, consistently or fast-paced? Or, will you vary your speed?

How quickly do you want to get there?

What are you willing to sacrifice in order to get there in the timeframe you desire (i.e., control, time, activities)?

What are you *not* willing to sacrifice that will need to be considered as part of your customized journey?

What control are you willing to give up or change?
What new skills or abilities are you willing to learn?

There is no 'right' answer to any of these questions. The answers are uniquely *yours.*

They're the ones you will follow because they are authentic and true for *you.*

Day 37

Psychology of Success: Model successful people.

Everything we aim to do has been done by someone else before us. We can simply break down their successful strategies and model (not necessarily copy exactly, but tailor to meet us) and follow a proven path, rather than "reinvent the wheel".

Modeling is a process that we have used our whole lives. It's the way we learned to stand and walk, the way we learned to talk, and the way we learned to do any of the millions of skills that we do automatically today.

What often happens when we are inspired to change and set off on a path of action toward our goals is that we immediately access all of the information that we've already gathered and look to others around us for additional support.

What if the information you have is NOT supportive of your goals?
What if those who attempt to help or those from whom you ask for help do not have any significant experience or mastery in what you're wanting to achieve?

"Don't base your decisions on the advice of those who don't have to live with your results."

When you embark on a change, know that many people will want to give you advice, it's simply human nature. Also know that *most* of that advice will be from people who don't know what they're talking about.
We can appreciate their intent, however it will help you to focus on the steps we share in this book and from professionals or from people who have already achieved the success you desire.

Principles vs. Practices

If we are to model other people's success, it is vital that we know what to model and how to do so. We must be able to distinguish **principles vs. practices.**

Think back to the success GPS. If you entered someone else's destination your road map will be right for *them*, not you. Maybe *what* to model from them was to simply use a GPS device.

The steps they took included entering their destination and hitting 'go'. This is the **practice** they took. A practice is specific and concrete, and is ideally the result of a guiding **principle**.

Principles are more fluid as they guide us through the many ways we can choose to accomplish things. Because there are many ways for you to take to achieve freedom, we can compare it to choosing one of the several routes that are often presented when you enter a destination on your GPS device.

Day 36

The 5 Steps That You Must Execute *Effectively* to Achieve Results That *Last*

To create results that last it is important to understand the 5-step psychological process that we all go through when approaching ANY goal or task.

It's not so much what you need to do in each of the 5-steps that is important, it's *how* you execute during each step that is key.

The technical term for this process is 'The Stages of Change Model', and it is a psychological sequence of events that occur in order for change to take place.

Our goal is to equip and empower you to make changes that last and understanding this model will help you to achieve both.

The model consists of 5 stages that we go through on the path to transformation (behavior change). Remember that you have the power to change your behavior at any time, in ways that can serve you positively or negatively. This is not a "one and done" process.

The majority of all diets fail because people go on them temporarily. They change their behavior in order to get results with the predetermined choice that they will go back to the behaviors that had them feeling depressed, lazy and unhealthy.

In order for the changes to stick we must let go of old habits and take on permanent new ones.

We are confident that by applying these principles and action steps you will create habits and make changes that you can keep for life.

By taking on the freedom mindset you can enjoy your lifestyle and whatever situations that it attracts.

This is true freedom and true self-control.

Stage 1: Pre-contemplation

The pre-contemplation stage occurs before any thought or awareness of change takes place. It typically occurs 6 months prior to the *beginning* of any change.
In this stage we are not even consciously considering change.
The need or desire for change may, however, be in our subconscious mind. If we are eating poorly or not exercising, for example, our subconscious mind is certainly aware of it!

Stage 2: Contemplation

Now we are consciously considering a change. We are aware of a difference in what we want and what we have. In this stage we weigh the pros and cons of staying the same or making the change. Only if we envision there being more cons to staying the same or more pros to change will we enter the next stage.

Stage 3: Preparation

In this stage we are gathering information and analyzing what it will take, what we have to do and how to take action. This is the research stage where we visit gyms for tours, read magazines, ask our friends, watch health-related shows, and look into equipment or the best home training program.
We still haven't taken any action toward changing our behavior, however we've gathered information in great detail about our options.

Stage 4: Action

This is the stage where we take action, from baby steps to giant leaps. As we go through this stage and work on our capabilities, we are only able to perform when we are applying conscious effort, taking actions toward our goals, living the way we know we need to live to become the person that we want to be.

In this stage you are working hard and it's paying off. You are feeling proud of yourself and it's getting noticed. People are commenting on how you look or noticing that you have a happier attitude.

Maybe you've had a few flirtatious glances from people at the coffee shop or on the way to work. Perhaps you've received compliments about an outfit that you've worn for a while, and you're feeling more noticed in general.

Keep Going! We graduate from this stage when we've made it to being unconsciously competent, when we can perform without consciously applying effort. It will be engrained in a way that is automatic. That is true Mastery!

But beware - at this action stage we need to be very alert, because this is the stage where ambivalence can occur. This is where we start to have mixed feelings about whether or not we want to continue on this change.

Occasionally this can occur because during the contemplation stage we did not consider enough the cons of staying the same and only focused on the pros of change - the "greener grass" we may have seen in someone else or in a dream scenario.

More often than not these wavering thoughts are due to an outside influence. Donut day at the office. Girls' night out. Date night. Your friends who don't want to change and secretly feel bad that you are doing so well. These are the saboteurs and they want to take you down!

To help you achieve success we need to be honest with you and prepare you for *all* situations so that you can be ready and have coping strategies in place (healthy ones that don't come in frozen pints).

Over the years we've seen these "negative nellies" come in the form of even your family or loved ones.
All too often has this brought on relationship breakdowns, ended friendships or caused alienation at work or in social circles.
Remember this - it's not about you. It's about them. Their demons, their weaknesses.
Any negative or destructive comments are all because they see *you* moving forward and it triggers *their* insecurities and fear.
Stay strong, focus more on the positive reactions that you are getting from others and most important the positive feelings you're having about yourself!

Stage 5: Maintenance

You've come so far and have taken small steps consistently enough that you've created new habits. Your simple actions led to habits, those habits became rituals and those rituals became part of your identity! You ARE transformed and now all you need to do is maintain that feeling, that view of yourself and the same mental (self) talk that helped you along the program.

If you're wondering what all of that is for you, keep reading as the subsequent chapters will literally reprogram your mind and create a new identity in line with the person you dream to be.

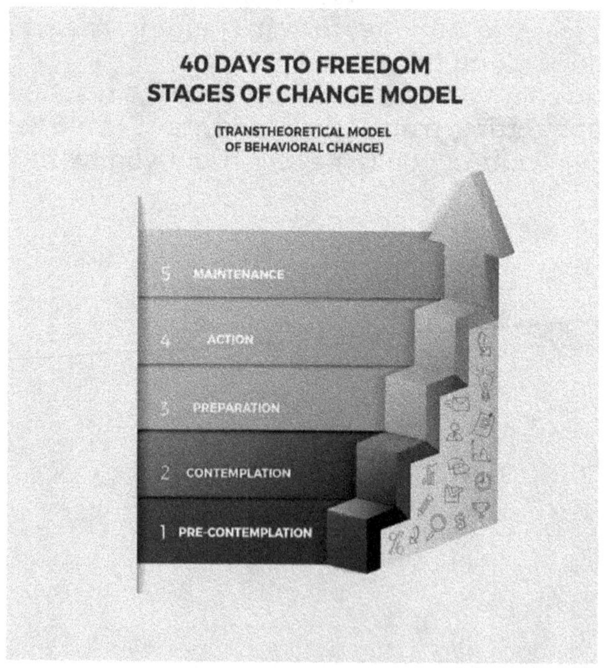

Putting this into action...
Consider this scenario as a way to illustrate that it's not so much what stage we go through or when, it's *how* we go through that stage and the intent, consciousness and awareness we bring to our time in each stage that makes **all** the difference.

'Lola' is building a house during summer. The weather is great and it's hot, so although the roof is incomplete, she feels no urgency to complete it.

Lola instead chooses to enjoy the present moment, not concerned with how the weather will change soon enough, or with the harsh rains and wind that typically come after summer.

Until the rains **do** come. Fast and hard!

Lola is forced in and out of pre-contemplation with the first few drops of rain, as the clouds begin to get heavy, dark and low.

The contemplation phase is accelerated through, as the rush is on to put up some kind of protection that will stop the rain from getting inside and ruining progress.

Preparation? Grab a nail, a hammer and *anything* that can be put up to keep the water out!

Her journey from Stage 1-Action occurs so fast that there is no chance for success.
The time, energy, focus and consciousness that is required for each stage hasn't happened, so the outcome is already doomed.

Add to that the fact that in the urgent action to *"just get something up to keep the rain out"*, her psychology is one of 'just-enough' and so the conscious - and subconscious - approach is that this is just *temporary*.

Consider how similar this is to someone's New Year's resolution.

Regardless of whether it is to lose weight, to get stronger, to learn a new skill or to start a new business, the fact that it is wrapped up in a package fit for the holidays all because we are about to enter into a new date sequence is what dooms it, just like the temporary roof.

With the changes of autumn and those of winter, this person is more focused on parties, feasts, and celebrations than looking good on the beach, and therefore the 'contemplation' of healthy eating, regular exercise and positive habits of health often get kicked to the curb.

This continues through the holiday period with all of the different activities and parties at work and at home or with children.

Suddenly it's Dec 28th and the New Year is around the corner. This person then accelerates through contemplation as they take a quick mental note of where they are physically, mentally, emotionally, financially, and so on.
If they come up short in any of those areas the guilt of months of inaction often ensues.

For this person, the next stage of '*Preparation*' consists of looking at what gym memberships may be on special, which new classes or Groupons friends are checking out, and hurriedly jumping into action... all the while knowing that their late preparation has laid the groundwork for only temporary results.

This unstable foundation is the reason why this person goes through cycles, never reaching the maintenance stage nor achieving long-term results.

Day 35

The Three Requisites for Change

In this book we identify three requisites for change.

1. **Release negative emotions or limiting beliefs & set a goal**
2. **Take action toward that goal**
3. **Maintain focus & consistency**

This book models those steps.

Most programs and most people skip step 1 and despite setting goals, focusing on what they want and building up as much frustration or motivation as possible to "take action", they run fast and hard into the brick wall of their negative emotions and limiting beliefs!

This hasn't worked for millions of others and it won't work for you... there is another way!

We are willing to break the paradigm of fitness, nutrition and weight loss books and invest all of the skills and tools we've learned over decades of successful clinical practice with thousands of clients to help you make this your 40 Days to Freedom, once and for all!

First, you must release negative emotions.

The primary negative emotions are:

a. Anger
b. Sadness
c. Fear
d. Hurt
e. Guilt

Yes, there may be others however they all "chunk up" into these negative umbrellas, if you will. Please take the time to think about and write down any of these emotions you have toward:

1. Your body (the way it looks from the outside)
2. Your self image
3. Your worthiness or being good enough
4. Past failures or inactions in the area of your health/fitness

Do you have any limiting beliefs in this area of your life?
Limiting beliefs are like heavy chains that tie you down and pull you back despite any positive intention or action to progress and move forward.

These beliefs will literally shape the world around you or your experience of it to sabotage and restrict you from success... because they want to be proven right, and your brain/ego wants to prove itself right more than any other goal you want. Being wrong, therefore, is more painful than the pain of feeling sick, feeling unworthy, feeling depressed, feeling disgusted at what you see in the mirror or even being judged or called names!

You MUST release these limiting beliefs in order for you to gain freedom, otherwise the results you achieve, if you are able to will yourself there, will disappear quickly because the fruits of your results are rooted in negativity and limitation.

"We cannot become what we want by remaining what we are!"

~ Max De Pree

In the areas of Health/Food/Body Image write down any past experiences or traumas that come up for you around the following emotions:

Anger

Toward yourself

Toward others

Feeling alone/abandonment

Sadness

Toward yourself

Toward others

Feelings that you want things to be different/
Feelings of grief or loss

Fear

Toward your future

Of what others may say/do/think/feel

Of failure or of success
(What may happen if things don't work out? What if things do work out and I can't handle it?)

Hurt

Toward yourself

Toward others

Specific traumas you've experienced related or unrelated to your body/image/health/freedom/control.

Guilt

Over your actions toward yourself

Over your actions toward others

Over inaction

Step 1 - Release these negative emotions and limiting beliefs.

Ben is a Master Practitioner in Mental & Emotional Release® Technique and Trainer in Time Line Therapy®, and has put together a guided release session to help you let go of these on your own.

Please visit
http://40DaysToFreedom.com/resources to gain access to this *guided release process* to do at home as often as necessary.

The best way to do this is with a trained professional. If you feel that the negative emotions or limiting beliefs are so deeply seeded please reach out to us to find a Master level practitioner in your area or to work directly with Ben.
Email **support@40DaysToFreedom.com**

PLEASE MAKE SURE THAT YOU GO THROUGH THE **RELEASING NEGATIVE EMOTIONS** PROCESS BEFORE PROGRESSING FURTHER WITH THIS BOOK

Next: You MUST Set A Goal

After releasing negative emotions, step 2 of the first requisite is to set a goal immediately following the release. You've created an empty container and the universe abhors a vacuum! If you do not fill it with a new positive intention and goal the old programming will seep back in.

Be aware that the quality of your goal and the motivator behind it will drastically *influence* or *infect* the journey and the outcome!

There are 2 types of motivators:

1. Positive Motivators
2. Negative Motivators

Have you ever wanted something so badly that you set a goal, took action, worked hard, even sacrificed to get it...and when you achieved it, it didn't give you the satisfaction you thought it would?

Did you think, "This doesn't taste/look/feel/sound as good as I imagined in my mind"?

This is likely because the whole time you were striving toward that goal you were operating from a negative motivator.

We call this a *move away from* rather than a *move toward* goal.

The Negative Motivator is what you **don't want** which is why you want to *move away from* it.

The Positive Motivator is what you **do want** and therefore you want to *move toward* it!

We've ALL used negative motivators. Sometimes they helped us to survive, get out of pain or even get some pleasure short-term.

Negative motivators can be very powerful short term, however they lose effect quickly, just as soon as the pain (causing the desire to move away from) disappears.

Some people have created a habit out of using negative motivators.

They constantly yo-yo above and below their happiness line (or weight line) by moving away from pain and then relaxing once they get some relief, only to drop themselves right back into pain because they didn't get themselves far enough out and *toward* something else.

Ben: *"I worked with a client who at 56 years old kept losing and gaining the same 10 lbs. over and over and over and over!*
At one point before we worked together she cut her calories down to 1200 per day, far too few and it was damaging her metabolism.

She kept yo-yoing from the urgency of the 'next event' to look good for, to the rebound of indulgence after it was over.

We worked together before her daughter's wedding and it all changed. She realized that she was moving away from looking bad in the short term at the next event rather than embracing a healthy body and lifestyle.

Once she let go of fear over calories and understood how to eat right for her body, she started to melt fat and look younger!"

In the next chapter, we'll reveal a way to empower yourself with Positive Motivators through the process of creating new beliefs, so that you can take powerful action toward your goal (the second requisite for change).

Day 34

The Process of Belief Creation

If beliefs can be formed in an instant, especially due to Significant Emotional Events, then can you agree that it's possible for you to re-create new ones that quickly? All you need is the right *recipe* for instant change.

If you follow the same pattern and create Significant Emotional Events intentionally, even if only within your mind, you can create the same instant change to support your desires!

How do you do this?

Make it Significant.
Focus on why freedom is important, what your WHY is for achieving it and the impact this will have on you. How would it affect your life, career, relationships, family, loved ones and the lives of so many others around you?

Remember when you wanted a material thing so badly that you thought it wasn't just going to be nice to have, it was a MUST-HAVE! You created only ONE potential outcome in your mind and that was that you'd have it.

Regardless of how long it took to save up the money, to wait for it to be ready or available, or how far you had to travel to get it, you were willing to do whatever it took because you placed so much SIGNIFICANCE on that thing or what having that thing would mean to you. This is what is possible for you to do with your freedom goals.

You'll need to choose to make them MUST-HAVES.

Make it Emotional.

Earlier we talked about *moving away from*, which is a negative motivator, and while it is a more powerful one short-term, it loses steam quickly.

Consider that when you have a powerful motivator to get out of a rut, you only feel that urge while you're *in* the rut, and as soon as you relieve the pain of being in it the motivator will quickly die.

For lasting change you want to focus on a positive motivator, a 'driver' if you will, that will not only move you toward your goal, but will accelerate and propel you there faster, easier and with so much force it will drive you *through* the finish line and beyond.

This is because the positive motivator never ends when you hit your target.

If your "move toward" is to be healthy and your goal is to be x lbs. and lean then the positive motivator of being healthy doesn't disappear when you achieve your desired short-term goal.

You simply move the goalposts and keep going because you can always achieve higher levels of health.

Suzanne's Story~

"For several years following the birth of my second child, I was significantly overweight and desperately fatigued. I was ignited to create a healthier lifestyle for myself and for my family when the pain of remaining the same- and being a poor role model for my children - exceeded the perceived pain of making a change.

While this was a negative motivator, it gave me the fuel to study, learn, dance and train my way to a healthy 40-pound weight loss. During that time, my motivation became increasingly positive as I realized my capabilities, changed my values and added supporting beliefs about myself. It was without question one of the most taxing yet cathartic and empowering years of my life.

It's incredible how much emotional baggage I dumped in my 36th year! The resulting transformation of my body, mind and 'being' ultimately attracted My Love and the genius behind this book, Ben Patwa.

Over the next few years together, we moved my goalposts several times to achieve higher fitness accomplishments using many of the principles and practices you'll learn in this book.

One of my proudest accomplishments within this arena to date was my deliberate and successful execution of a Significant Emotional Event (S.E.E.) to break through long-held limiting beliefs about my worthiness to be seen and heard as a strong voice in women's health and empowerment.

My fear of the limelight and especially the stage further served to stifle the voice that already struggled to emerge, having wrestled with shyness most of my life.

At the age of 40, I decided to boldly face my fear of the stage and compete in my first fitness competition. There were few things more terrifying to me at the time than to elect to traipse across a fluorescent stage wearing a tiny bikini and stilettos in front of a judgmental crowd.

This scenario challenged all that I believed myself to be. It scolded the young Christian schoolgirl cowering in the corner of my mind. It sneered at the mother who dared to risk tainting her daughter's perception of her own healthy body image, and threatened to show support for the distasteful projection of what I thought this choice of 'exposure' was perpetuating in women's fitness.

Confident in my ability to continue to gracefully cultivate my intended ongoing message and healthy modeling for my daughter, and holding a clear vision of my overarching goal of self-improvement so I could better serve others, I committed to doing whatever it took. I needed to expose myself, literally and figuratively.

By creating positive associations with supportive people and environments, and by studying NLP, I was able to replace my fear and apprehension with confidence, and took 2nd place in the competition! I had now earned the recognition and platform I desired to fulfill my dream to help women feel empowered in health and fitness! I now embrace the 'stage' and I am proud of the example I am for my daughter!

Day 33

Placing Success In Your Future

The third requisite for change is to maintain focus & consistency. So now we will help you to stay on track in moving toward your goal.
We will give you a vision of what success will look, feel and sound like so it becomes a path to follow.

Think of your future.

What are some of the emotions that you will feel now that you've achieved freedom?
Close your eyes (once you've finished reading this of course) and imagine yourself having already achieved the goal.

Go forward into the future and see yourself after successfully completing your 40 Days to Freedom.

Looking back on the timeline, notice what you see, hear, and feel now that you've totally succeeded and even surpassed all expectations for yourself!

Ready, go...

Go to **http://40DaysToFreedom.com/resources** for online video of timeline session and guided instruction.

Journal about this experience.

Day 32

Who do you want to be?

In our experience with working with clients over the years, perhaps the #1 issue that causes pain for people is the difference between their current reflection and the image they have in their mind of who they truly are (ego image).

Consider someone who suffers from Anorexia. He/she has an extreme difference between their interpretation of their current image, which they see as very fat, and the image the rest of the world sees as dangerously thin. This is called "Body Image Distortion".

While they set out to lose more and more weight in pursuit of a body that is, to them, acceptable in size, they will never achieve happiness AND a healthy body without changing the internal image of themselves and re-calibrating how they look in the mirror and what they see (or think they see).

So if there can be only one "you", in your reflection and in your mind, who do you want to be?

What do you know you need to do that you're not doing?
(Let these become your initial action steps because you are already convinced that you need to do them).

Power State - When you are seeing and feeling your ideal version of yourself, what is present then that is not present now?
(This is what to *start* doing).

Stuck State - When you are not being the ideal version of yourself, what is NOT present then that IS present now?
(This is what to *stop* doing).

These questions help you to create boundaries and to protect your new identity level.

Who are you?
Who are you not?

These are some of the most powerful questions because the answers drive our beliefs about others and ourselves. Our beliefs determine our values. Our values influence our behavior. Our behavior creates our results - those we want and those we don't want.

Once we realize that we truly create all of the results in our lives, *even those we want to blame others for*, we can realize results that last a lifetime.

Our decisions revolving around who we are and who we are not will become very clear. Black and White. Yes or No. We become strong, decisive, powerful, and clear which leads to peace, happiness and most important, Freedom.

Would you like cake?
"I don't eat cake."
Compare this to "Oh, that looks delicious, *BUT* I can't/shouldn't eat cake."

What sounds more powerful to you?

Whoever you choose to be, the internal identity of you HAS to be in alignment with your external habits, actions and lifestyle for you to be happy and maintain your results/ideal self.

***Self-mastery is knowing how much of any of the above you can be while still maintaining an integrity (meaning keeping it all together) along your path (meaning that you still get to your destination).**

This is our "**double mirror**" process.

Imagine if you set out to drive your car 100 mph for 1000 miles... and only put in 3 gallons of gas, didn't replenish the oil or consider the temperature gauge... you *probably* wouldn't make it, right?

We must consider the same details for ourselves. We have a *range* of how fast we can go before we need a rest, how hot we can burn and how much fuel we need.

Gas pumps have a really cool feature, the part that "clicks" to shut off the gas flow when your tank is full so that you don't overflow and spill flammable liquid all over you and your car.

We need to remember that we also have one of these, our gut brain, yet many of us have lost connection to it, possibly because it doesn't make a loud click and shudder.
Instead it sends an internal sensation telling us when we've had enough to eat. It tells us when we've eaten the right and the wrong foods and it gives us feedback to let us know when we're on the right track.

Imagine if you were in a relationship where the connection had broken down so badly that whenever you communicated something important the other person ignored you, or even worse blatantly violated your request. You would probably stop talking, right?

Well the same reaction happens in our bodies! If your gut tells your brain what it needs and yet it doesn't get it, things break down. If the gut tells the brain that what is being consumed is harming the body and it keeps happening, the gut will simply stop making the effort to communicate.

We need to repair the relationship so that we can listen and trust what is being communicated! Until that happens, "going with your gut" and believing that you don't have a negative reaction to certain foods is reckless.

How do we repair the relationship? Read on...

It takes the body 4-7 days to completely metabolize and cleanse any food (or drug). We utilize a very easy and free test to identify food sensitivities, addictions and reactions.

It's called a 7-day elimination test.

We invite you to come off of a food that you want to test or a food you think you can't do without, or especially a food you *don't* think has control over you that you eat frequently.

Simply cut this food out of your diet for 7 days and take note of how you feel during the process.
(Go to **http://40DaysToFreedom.com/resources** for our sample 4-day test diet and specialized diet record sheets to help you get more clear on how you Respond to different foods).

What will happen may shock you.
By the 4th day you will experience one of two things:

1. You will feel a huge craving for the food that you cut out, so much so that you may experience symptoms of "cold turkey" such as mental fog, hunger, and aggression.

2. You may experience the absence of "The Voices". "The Voices" is a term we give to those craving conversations that go on in our client's heads. They differ from our intuition or our gut brain's messages of what we really need.

Additional recommendations:

Just as you would use a cast to help a broken bone, we recommend that you use these supplements during your rehabilitation phase to help you to begin to repair your gut.

Our Gut Repair Formula:

- Glutamine Blend with specific prebiotics
- High power Probiotics

These 2 supplements seem to have a positive effect on the environment in your gut, thereby improving function and silencing "The Voices".

Day 31

Your Abusive Relationship

Are you in an abusive relationship, where you are both the victim AND the abuser?

Consider the relationship that you have with food.

Do you use food to influence your feelings?

Do you use food to change a state that you are in?

Do you use food to create a more pleasurable experience?

Do you find yourself craving a certain food or type of food if you've not had it for a few days?

Do you notice a difference in your mood if you have or haven't had a certain food recently?

Do *others* notice if you haven't eaten a certain food in a while?

Do you have friends who would say that you love a certain food because they know it'll make you feel happier?

If you answered 'Yes' to any of these questions then you may have a relationship to food that is similar to that of a drug.

Remember, our dependent relationship to food often wasn't created by us. It was created long before we had complete control over what we consumed.

Long before we started to make our own choices, spend our own money and manage our own feelings, food was used to influence and control us.

Do you have an abusive relationship with your mind?

If you spoke to someone else the way you speak to yourself in your head, would they be your friend?

Would they support you through thick and thin?

Would they love you unconditionally and accept you in all ways?

Plan for tomorrow, today!

When you make a specific plan for a day the night before, you can go to sleep and allow your unconscious mind to navigate all of the necessary things you need to do. You can consider different scenarios and potential obstacles, all in your sleep.

It's like 6-8 hours of mental rehearsal for your day ahead!

This is why we plan for tomorrow, today. We set two kinds of goals, and to be successful over the long haul we need BOTH.

These two kinds of goals can be classified as *AIM* goals and *END* goals.

***AIM* goals NEVER END.**
They serve as a guiding light to follow, and stay active until *you* choose to change them (which rarely happens because they are linked to your values).
An example of an AIM goal is "to be healthy and vital". Can you see how this never ends?

***END* goals are meant to END.**
For example if we have an end goal to lose 10 lbs. it *ends* when 10 lbs. have been lost, otherwise if we kept losing 10 lbs. over and over we would wither away and die.

Look back and see if you've ever felt an inner turmoil around achieving your goals or if you've felt "split" inside, with part of you wanting the end goal and part of you wanting *more* than simply the result.

Have you ever set a goal, worked your butt off to achieve it and when you finally get it, you're left feeling "is that it?!"

Ben: *"I had a client early on in my career who was VERY motivated by money and wanted to buy himself a Porsche.*

I've always been skilled at asking questions to help someone identify their inner connections to feelings and what is driving them, so we quickly discovered that he would feel 'proud' and 'worth something' by owning it.

With a few more precise questions we established that these were two feelings that he had never felt from his father growing up, and realized that he was simply chasing the goal to prove something to himself (which was really to prove to his dad).

Despite this realization he still stayed committed to his goal (an END goal) pushing and pushing, shaping his choices, time and energy...and what happened when he finally bought his Porsche?

He drove it for a few months, feeling great. Proud. Worth something. Then it wore thin, and he realized that it was in his words, 'just a car'."

You see, he placed all of his worth and pride in what he *thought* the Porsche would give him, when the real issue was the void he was trying to fill.

The tragedy of life does not lie in not reaching your goal. The tragedy lies in having no goals to reach.

~ Benjamin Mays

Two sides to the coin.

To begin to fill the gap between where you are and where you want to be we will need an approach that considers the *two* sides of the coin.

On one side we have all of the negative factors, those things that are like taking steps backward, away from our goal. These are the thoughts, feelings and actions that we need to stop doing or do less.

We see people take this approach often when they are in desperation, feeling the *need* to reach their goal, and often when they feel as though time is running out on them.

Consider the woman who has just realized that her vacation to a hot, sunny beach is less than 2 weeks away and she has left it far too late to get into shape the way she promised herself when she booked the trip.

With this sense of urgency, she feels desperate. She has seen all of the images on the website and in the magazines that show all of the people will be in great shape, and now she is feeling ashamed of her body and angry with herself for not getting started early enough.

Fueled with negative emotions and a desire to *move away* from embarrassment and shame, she attempts to cut out as many foods and calories as she can. She stops all alcohol and goes on a sugar-free diet.

She tells her friends what she has decided to do and lets them know that they can't tempt her with their lifestyle choices so they will either need to adjust or stay away until after her trip.

The other side of the coin has the positive factors, those things that lead us *toward* our desired outcome.

They are the thoughts, feelings and actions we need to start doing or do more!

It is the approach of combining *both* sides of the coin that creates massive, lasting change.

All too often we see someone attempt to play one side of the coin based on the strongest emotion at the time, either cutting things out due to *moving away* from a negative result, or adding things in as they *move toward* a desired result.

If you only stop doing things that pull you in the wrong direction you will only stop yourself from sinking deeper. What you won't do is move yourself at all in the *right* direction.

If you only attempt to start doing things that drive you toward your goal without stopping the negative factors then it's like driving down the road with one foot on the gas *and* one foot on the brake!

CONGRATULATIONS!

You've just completed the first 10 Days!

This was all about leading you through the pre-contemplation, contemplation and preparation stages of change.

Next...
We spring into **ACTION** with our focused 30-day countdown to transform your habits, mindset, body image and relationship to food.

As Abraham Lincoln said,

"Give me 6 hours to chop down a tree and I'd spend the first 4 sharpening the axe."

40 Days To Freedom
Transformation Fitness Program

As you progress through the next 30 days you will find all of the tips you need to take action and maintain focus on your goal to freedom.

If you would like more support or to take your results up a notch, we have a complete 30-day fitness program that goes hand-in-hand with the steps in this book.

You'll receive daily emails, video guides, exercise programs with instruction on correct form as well as nutrition guidelines and recipes to help you take the steps to freedom *together* instead of alone.

One of the major benefits of the program is the Facebook group where you will receive support, motivation, accountability and answers to all of your questions.

Here is a Success Story from one of the graduates of our program...

"I was ready to make a change in my lifestyle with a program that I could incorporate into my daily routine and for the rest of my life.

I had been feeling down on myself because I had put on 15 pounds and had lost the motivation to work out.

When I found this program, I was very excited to get started because I knew it was something I could stick to.

It's very tough to say which part was my favorite because the entire program was enjoyable.

For starters I found the website to be very easy to navigate. It was very organized! Ben and Suzanne did an amazing job of creating recipes, shopping lists and downloadable nutrition guidelines.

The recipes are easy to follow and most important very tasty...at no point on this journey did I feel deprived of anything!

I loved the workout routines because I was able to print out the daily exercises and review the videos before hitting the gym. While at the gym I would often view the videos again before I did the exercise to make sure I had the right form.

I believe that the most beneficial part to me was the support from the private Facebook page. Other participants as well as Ben and Suzanne gave encouragement, suggestions, and support. They were always there to answer any questions I had.

Throughout the 30 days I lost a total of 15 pounds and I have never felt so great! My allergies went away, I find myself sleeping better, and my energy is through the roof."

~ Adriana S.

Day 30

Public Declaration of Independence

We started with goals and now we invite you to make a powerful declaration. A powerful first ACTION.

Think of this as a 'line in the sand' as a symbol or declaration of your decision to make this program work, for you to make the *freedom lifestyle* work.

This is your **Public Declaration of Independence**!

We ask you to make it known publicly that you are taking control of your mind, body and health with these steps toward freedom. Something very powerful happens when you do this. You see, the mind and the ego wants to keep us "safe" and that includes emotionally safe.

When we are considering a change, our minds and our egos often tell us to "play it safe" in order to limit the disappointment if we don't succeed. When we publicly declare our commitment however, now our minds and egos want for us to succeed so that we don't fall flat on our faces.

For this to work effectively though we must set it up in a way to find and knock out the saboteur.

The saboteur is the part of you that wants you to fail, the part that thinks you don't really know what you want and that you'll be happier if you just stay the same.

1) Write a public declaration of independence.

Share this publicly in as many places as you can.

- Tell your friends, colleagues and family.
- Post on social media.
- Share it within our private forum.

DECLARE YOUR COMMITMENT TO FREEDOM!

Please use:

#40DaysToFreedom
#PublicDeclarationOfIndependence when posting.

Keep this on display in your house.
On the refrigerator and/or in your bedroom are good places.

If you have a vision board you can pin this up on there too.

If you don't have a vision board you can watch a video about how to create one on our resource page.

http://40DaysToFreedom.com/resources

2) Write a breakup letter to Mr./Ms. Saboteur. This will formalize your separation and anchor the experience for you.

“Dear Mr./Ms. Saboteur,

I no longer tolerate...

You have cost me...

I commit to...

I deserve...

I am free without you.”

Signed & dated

Day 29

Twenty years from now you will look back more regretfully upon the things you didn't do than those you did. So set free the bowlines, sail away from safe harbor. Dream. Explore. Discover.

- Mark Twain

Today's mindset to adopt is one of the beginner, the action-taker, one who starts something.
There is pure excitement, eagerness and optimism that fuels someone into action, sometimes even prematurely, and this is the perfect mindset for today.

You are embarking on a journey where you can clearly see what you're leaving behind, having been there before. You may not be able to clearly see or fully grasp what you'll be moving into, however. This takes trust.

Think of this as similar to being on the shores of a familiar coastline and casting your boat into the water. You are very clear about what you're leaving. The firm solid ground you now call home, the familiarity of what you know.

Looking out into the ocean that spans further than you can see, you are unsure about what lies ahead and what you may encounter along the way yet this is the canvas of complete opportunity for you to create your future!

If you never set sail because you were waiting to see the destination *before* you took action, then you may never get to experience the soft sand of the beach, the luscious trees with delicious fruits, and the breathtaking views of the new land you'll call home.

This book is all about your mind and so we are going to play some tricks on it to help you get started. Have you ever noticed how most nutrition or weight loss books and programs focus immediately on what to "cut out" of your life?

In our experience this is a recipe for disaster because it traps you in a cycle of restriction and attributes most success to a "less than" or *move away from* lifestyle.

Our goal is to create freedom, and therefore we intend to add so much goodness to your mind, body, and to your plate that you will naturally release or let go of the choices that sabotage or hold you back.

Consider the person who wants to quit smoking. They can try with all of their willpower and focus on the benefits of giving up however as soon as stress kicks in with issues at work, struggles in relationships, or simply an aggressive driver, they will default back to a habit that they know gives them immediate, if short-lived, relief.

When this same person quits smoking and replaces that vice with something else, hopefully a healthier one, they will default to the new habit whenever their life hits a bump in the road.

This program is all about releasing what doesn't work and replacing that with positive, supportive and productive actions and habits.

Reinforce with supplementation or additional lifestyle adjustments for rapid success and sustained results, which includes you becoming equipped and empowered to do so.

Start your Freedom Journal

Each day we invite you to journal your progress. Some days we will prompt you with questions. Other days we will invite you to document your key wins, breakthroughs or insights along your journey as these can be powerful reinforcers for you.

Journal Questions

These journal questions are a powerful start to your awareness practice.
Have you ever bought a car, a dress, or a pair of shoes and soon thereafter saw the very thing you bought everywhere you went?
That is because our brains filter the 126 pieces of information most relevant to us and place them in our conscious mind.

The rest (approximately 11 billion pieces of information per second) that we take in through our 5 senses gets distorted, deleted or generalized. This can lead to a skewed reality or memory of what *really* happened along our journey and that is a great reason to journal each day/night.

Let's start with some questions that will help you to gain leverage over your past way of doing things. You are smart, you have experience and you are capable of greatness.

What may also be present is the habit of inaction or procrastination (also resistance) to the things that you know you need to do and the creation (distortion) of a theory that you need to learn or find something that you don't already have in order to get the results you desire.

Take some time to answer these questions with as much rich detail, vulnerability and truth as you can. We suggest that you answer journal questions as you are now, rather than as you used to be, want to be or think you should be.
Any time we want you to do something different we will explain and guide you through that as a process.

What do you know that you need to cut out that you haven't cut out yet?

What do you know you need to start doing and haven't started doing yet?

What environmental factors cause you to struggle with sticking to your goals and dreams?

What people act as saboteurs or negative drains on your energy and progress?

The more clarity and awareness you have around these factors the more empowered you are to make conscious choices and the more free you become.

Day 28

Never start work before breakfast, if you do have to work before breakfast, eat breakfast first.

- Josh Billings

From today forward, increase your breakfast size.

If you usually eat nothing, eat something.
If you eat donuts, please skip the donuts, and add protein!

Our primary focus here is blood sugar stabilization. Our invitation is for you to gain control of your glucose regulation, or the way that your blood sugar fluctuates throughout your day.

Increasing the size of your breakfast starts your insulin rise and fall on a much more gradual basis rather than the extreme roller coaster that can happen with a small or no-breakfast start to the day. How does this happen?

If you start the day primarily with coffee, a stimulant, and/or bread-based foods like pastries/toast/bagels then that spikes your insulin, which is a hormone responsible for removing sugar from your bloodstream.

Dump copious amounts of sugar into your bloodstream first thing in the morning and you're spiking insulin to a peak like Everest... What comes after such a sudden extreme high? Insulin drops like one of Muhammad Ali's opponents.

When we add protein we are adding a food source, which is much harder to break down. What this does is buffer the spike in insulin keeping it much smoother and more consistent over the day.

Because protein takes a lot longer to break down it gives us a feeling of being full sooner and for a longer period of time, and this can help dramatically in stabilizing your appetite and overcoming food cravings.

What you'll find is that many sweet cravings that happened later in the evening are because you didn't get enough protein earlier in the day, leaving you at the mercy of the “glucose roller coaster”.

Here’s your invitation today: Eat **More**!

Continue eating the same diet that you would normally eat for an entire day and just bulk up the amount of protein that you have for breakfast and we are confident that by the end of the day you'll feel more in control of your food cravings.

Some examples of how you can increase your protein intake for breakfast are:

- Add two strips of organic, nitrate free, gluten-free bacon to your breakfast meal. Yes... Bacon!

- Eat two whole, sunny side up, pasture raised eggs

- Have a few ounces of grass-fed beef steak, thinly sliced

- If you struggle with appetite in the morning or simply have a habit of running late out of the door then you can try drinking a protein shake instead.

We recommend high-quality grass-fed whey protein powder and grass-fed meat sources on our website or you can find others online or at your local high-end supermarket.

Go to **http://40DaysToFreedom.com/resources** for one of our favorite protein shake recipes for breakfast!

Journal Questions

How have you taken more action in these past 3 days than you have in past?

What's one WIN that you've already had since starting this book?

What is one insight about yourself that you've gained since starting?

Day 27

In life, what more can you ask for but to be real? To fulfill one's potential we have great works ahead of us, and it needs devotion and much energy!

~ Bruce Lee

Energy Drains.

Consider where your time and energy drains are in your current lifestyle.

Often people struggle to fit everything they want to do, or feel they need to do, into the day.
When we examine how they spend that day, and where they place their time, energy and focus it is clear to see areas where they could restructure and find plenty of time to take action.

Some of the more obvious energy drains are TV, Facebook, email, sleeping in, taking a nap and so many more.

It can be human nature to overestimate how long it may take to achieve something, or to anticipate that there will be more obstacles than may actually show up.

"I've had a lot of worries in my life, most of which never happened."

- Mark Twain

What happens is that you'll end up waiting for a perfect situation or the perfect time to show up, and potentially wait so long that you end up never making a move at all.

This is analogous to attempting to throw a ball 30 ft. and only feeling ready when you can do that in *one* shot.

What if you threw the ball 5 ft., followed up and threw it another 5 ft., and so on? Where would you be compared to the version of you who is still attempting to throw the ball 30 ft. in *one* shot?

What would it mean to you, if you made it 30 ft. in six tosses vs. one? Would the destination be any different?

Consider where you are draining your own energy by *needing* your life and the situations you face to be a certain way.

Take a close look at your day and see if you are passing up a 30-minute opportunity waiting for a 60-minute window.

Look to find an extra 30 minutes per day. It may just change your life.

Journal Questions

Many people create short-term goals at the mercy of others, for example they focus on earning money in the short term and push their health or fitness out to the future.

"When I complete x then I'll be able to focus on y."

Today consider:

What goals or dreams have you been putting off for a future date?

What have you been waiting for, before you'll start? (Permission, everything to be right, "when I have the money, time, skills, etc.")

Day 26

Do something today that your future self will thank you for!

On Day 28 we recommended that you *add* more food to your plate. Today we invite you to *release* draining foods.

If you consume **sodas, gluten, energy drinks or alcohol** then we recommend that you commit to releasing those now, if only to prove to yourself that you *are* capable of doing it and that you *are* in control of your consumption.

Consider that each of these foods or drinks cause incredibly drastic chemical changes in your body when you consume them.

Soda: The majority of all sodas contain High Fructose Corn Syrup. When you realize that Fructose is the most fattening substance to the human body it is obvious why we have seen the expanding waistlines of populations around the world, especially where a certain heavily marketed brand has shown up.

Gluten: When you consume gluten it is highly likely that you are *not* chewing on a raw sheath of wheat or nibbling on the whole grains. Instead you are probably chowing down on something that was made from flour.

Pasta, Pizza, bread, bagels, cookies, sauces, fillers in prepared meats, soups - this stuff is everywhere!

Let's look at what that flour does when it hits your gut...

When a grain is milled into flour, the surface area increases by 10,000 times. That means that it is absorbed 10,000 times faster than the natural grain would when consumed.

This creates a huge spike in insulin, your storage hormone, which opens your fats cells for storage and actually *decreases* your ability to burn fat. If there is a single hormone that is responsible for weight gain and lethargy, it's insulin.

Think about this the next time you go to reach for some flour-y carbohydrate on its own (crackers, for example).

Watch our video on effects of combining fats & carbohydrates on the resource page – 40DaysToFreedom.com/resources

If this isn't enough of a reason to *go against the grain* and cut them all out completely, try these gluten-free grains as substitutes:

1. Corn (GMO-free, if you can find it)
2. Millet
3. Buckwheat
4. Rice – brown or basmati
5. Quinoa (actually a seed, but substitutes nicely)

Please remember that you'll be eating these in the form of flour too though, so be sure to combine them with the increased protein you added from yesterday.

Energy drinks: The use of synthetic stimulants has become a huge craze in the lives of highly stressed corporate executives and athletes of all arenas, especially thanks to slick advertising, attractive branding and appealing sponsorships.

What is potentially more worrying to see is the high numbers of mothers resorting to energy drinks to keep up with busy schedules, young children running at their ankles and the nearly full-time job of family chauffeur.

College students and even high school students are using energy drinks or consuming coffee "blended" drinks to help them through cramming, exams and increased workloads.

What all of these individuals may not understand is that the stimulants in these energy drinks and the concentrated potency are thrashing their thyroid and adrenal glands. Considering how many younger women are developing thyroid cancers, hormone imbalance and adrenal fatigue it seems clear that the very drinks they are grabbing for a "short-term boost" may be leading to long-term burn out!

Alcohol: Alcohol is one of the most quickly absorbed things you can consume! It gets sucked right through the stomach wall and doesn't need to go into the small intestine like most other foods. This is why we see many medicines in an alcohol solution, to help us absorb the medicine into our blood faster.

What consuming alcohol can do is pull undigested food particles into your bloodstream in the same way! When this happens, our immune system gets stimulated as if there was an invader and the white blood cells start attacking the food as if it were harmful.

This is the process by which we develop food sensitivities, and while alcohol is a primary contributor to this phenomenon, it is one substance of many possible culprits. This is why it is very important to check for food intolerances if you are not getting the results that your effort deserves.

If you are eating copious amounts of sugar, starchy carbs and grains and getting no exercise then it is a simple equation why you may not be in an optimal body shape. This equation looks like 2 + 2 = 4.

When you *are* working out, watching what you eat and attempting to make the best choices you can and *still* aren't getting results - that's an anomaly and this may require more testing to help you get to the root of the issue.
This equation looks more like 2 + 2 = *not* 4.

We simplify this by saying
"If 2 + 2 does not = 4, then you have a problem".

We share more about testing options near the end of this book (p. 211) and on our resource page.
Look for
"If you're not assessing, you're guessing"
at **http://40DaysToFreedom.com/resources**

We also highly recommend that you add a few supplements to aid in the process of tolerating the initial effects you'll feel from changing your diet over the course of the next few weeks.

Why?
There is considerably less nutrition in food today than there was just 100-200 years ago.

The introduction of chemical farming has drastically reduced the quality and availability of nutrients and has made it necessary to support our bodies with high quality supplementation.

Not all supplements are created equal however, and we advise against using grocery store or chain pharmacy brands, as these have often been found not to contain what is promised on the label.

The New York Times recently published an article revealing that the New York Attorney General's office found that after conducting tests on products of four national retailers, they were found to either contain *none* of the herbal ingredients listed on the label or had *unlisted* fillers such as legumes or wheat (potentially harmful for those with sensitivities or allergies) even though the bottles included guarantees not to contain those allergens!

The supplements to consider adding to your regime right away are

- **5-HTP,**
- **Digestive Enzymes,**
- **L-Tyrosine,**
- **Fish Oil, and**
- **Probiotics.**

For video explanations of each of these supplements, how they work and why we recommend them as well as a supplement guide and where to source high-quality formulations,
please visit **http://40DaysToFreedom.com/resources**

Day 25

You won't regret the junk food you don't eat today, tomorrow.

Don't starve through the day to binge at night.

We have worked with professional ballet dancers and athletes who gorge on pints of ice cream and bags of candy each evening and struggle to gain control of their eating.

Why would this happen to such disciplined people?

We call it unsustainable eating.
They go all day limiting calories and restricting what and how they eat, only to come home exhausted and binge on sugary foods.

The sour part is how out of control they feel.
How could they regain control?

We offer a general solution, however we believe that everyone is different and requires a customized approach. To find out more about our customized programs visit
http://40DaysToFreedom.com/resources.

Our general solution is the *top down* approach:

Eat your largest meal in the morning.
Decrease the portion size of each subsequent meal so that your smallest meal is the last meal of your day, around one hour before bed.

This can also be referred to as the upside-down triangle (rather than pear) model. Your body will follow suit as it transforms with a V-shape torso narrowing to a slim waist.

Eat your meals from small to large and you'll end up looking like that pear!

Journal Questions

Where have you been living in an unsustainable way in your life?

What have you been hiding from others as a dirty little secret?
For many of our athlete clients it was nighttime binging on candy. Challenge yourself to go deep and identify what is really hiding in your shadow.

We suggest that you write this on a blank sheet of paper, and should you wish, ceremoniously burn it in a safe place of course.

Day 24

When people undermine your dreams, predict your doom or criticize you, remember that they are telling you *their* story, not yours.

Avoid/limit unsupportive people and environments.

Today you may have friends, family, colleagues and work relationships with people that take more from your progress than they support it.
While the changes we're advising may be daunting, your future self will thank you for the courage and proactive steps you take today to limit how much you have them in your environment.

If you were to classify people into 2 categories,

1. Those that **in**fect you
2. Those that **af**fect you

Where would the people in your day-to-day life fall? Are you willing to let go of what you have for what you want?

Today's action step is all about creating, intentionally and consciously, a positive, supportive environment, not only for this journey, but for your life as a whole.

As Dr. Bruce Lipton shares in his work "*Biology of Belief*" our health is more greatly impacted by our environment than our genetics.

This implies that any disease processes or ill health we experience has more to do with who we are around, the locations and situations we put ourselves in and how those environments affect us, than our genetic makeup or what we've inherited from our parents.

Seize control of your life today by controlling or managing your environment.

There may be situations that you place yourself in by default or automatic pilot rather than conscious intent. We will help you uncover those.

On the next page please take time to answer the questions in the spaces provided or continue to fill out your personal Freedom Journal.

I will not let anyone walk through my mind with their dirty feet.

- Mahatma Gandhi

Journal Questions

Where do I go on a daily basis that uplifts and inspires me?

Where do I go on a daily basis than drains or depletes me?

Who do I surround myself with that uplifts and inspires me?

Who do I surround myself with that drains or depletes me?

If I could add someone or somewhere to my life that would support my progress and desired lifestyle, who or where would that be?

Day 23

Time and health are two precious assets that we don't recognize and appreciate until they have been depleted.

~ Denis Waitley

We're one week in!
Congratulations, as you have hit a significant milestone.

New habits take 7-21 days to form so you are now in the transformation phase and each step you take in the direction of your goal serves to reinforce the new pattern and distance you from your old ones.

What's your health $/hr?

You know how some of us clock in and clock out at work? What if we kept that kind of record for our lives?

Where do you spend your time daily, weekly or monthly?
Would you continue to do that if you had to spend money instead of time?

If we asked you to put a $ amount on your time what would you say?

Most people would default to their work wage, or what they charge for their top services.
If we were to ask someone close to dying, they would probably answer very differently.

Ben: I have two movie recommendations for you, and these are part of your homework.
The first is a classic and award-winning movie; the second is more for comedic and dramatic effect.

1. Scent of a Woman. This is one of my favorite movies for many reasons and has numerous stellar scenes from Al Pacino. He goes from feeling sorry for himself because he went blind in the war, to choosing to take his own life as way to stop the pain. It wasn't until he witnessed the innocence and purpose of a young boy and was

forced into a leadership role to protect him from the bureaucracy of a private school that he realized the preciousness of his life through others. He realized how sacred integrity and honor were to him and got the feeling of being alive again through contribution.

2. If you haven't seen the movie "Bucket List" with Jack Nicholson and Morgan Freeman I highly recommend it. Now it's not going to 'wow' you for originality or for best script of the year, however it might help open your mind to the choices we make and what we consider to be priority and what we take for granted (often until it's too late).

Ben: *"When I was 18 I almost lost my life when both of my kidneys failed and I had to have an emergency operation. Please take it from me and the young, superhuman version of me back then, who thought that I had centuries of time on this planet... I don't.*

None of us are getting out of life alive, so we might as well make the most of it!"

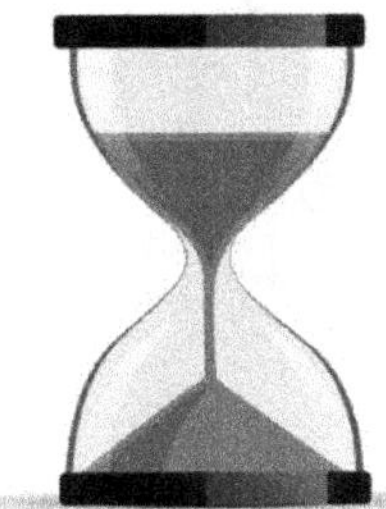

This may be a crucial time to consider what value you place on the dwindling sand in the hourglass of your life. - Ben Patwa

Journal Questions

It is clear that having someone other than yourself to live and fight for gives us a heroic and almost superhuman quality/strength.

Consider the stories of a grandmother who lifted a car to free a young child, or the conditions people endure to save others up on Mount Everest.

If you were to realize that your life has a purpose for others, who would be in your corner?

Who would you be fighting for, getting healthy for and going through pain and effort for?

Day 22

The measure of who we are is what we do with what we have.

~ Vince Lombardi

We are what we absorb.

We've talked a lot about reducing our exposure to negative/toxic people. You have placed a value on your time, your energy and your life. This is controlling your environment and what you absorb from it.

Now let's talk food.

You've probably heard or read the saying "You are what you eat". Well that isn't entirely true. It isn't so much based on what we put in our mouths, as it is what we absorb from what we eat. Specifically, it's the nutrients we absorb and can use.

Starting today we recommend that you add one of our Freedom Formula pillars to your daily routine.

Digestive enzymes.

Please remember that not all foods are created equal and studies have shown that the nutrient levels of inorganic (conventional) foods are significantly lower than those of organic. The argument isn't whether organic foods are some form of "superfood". They are what nature's normal used to be. The argument is that inorganic foods are so depleted that they often *take* more from your body than they give!

In addition to this, the majority of vitamins and minerals that your body needs to absorb are **fat-soluble**. Yes, that fatty stuff that so many people fear is actually responsible for helping you to absorb most of your nutrients!

We recommend a high quality digestive enzyme blend that works in acidic and alkaline environments to help you digest fats, proteins and carbohydrates to absorb maximum nutrition.

Today, also **add extra raw fats** to a few of your meals or snacks throughout the day, and for the rest of the week.
Good choices to choose from are (pick 2 per day):

- ¼ teaspoon of coconut oil eaten raw or on top of veggies
- 1 teaspoon of organic almond butter twice per day
- ½ avocado with a meal, or blended in a shake
- Make your own salad dressings with extra virgin olive oil
- “Emergency nut supply” (zip lock bag some nuts and stash them everywhere!

(Go to **http://40DaysToFreedom.com/resources** for our recommendations and for our favorite homemade salad dressing recipe!)

Journal Questions

Why is this transformation important to you?

What would it bring into your life once you've shown yourself that you can see this through?

Where have you settled for comfort when you could have had excellence, greatness and your wildest dreams all at once?

Day 21

Every positive change in your life begins with a clear, unequivocal decision that you are going to either do something or stop doing something.

~ Brian Tracy

This is your breakthrough day!

Clinically we've seen that clients who have cut out foods, drugs, habits or experiences that they were addicted to took 4-7 days to "break free".
You've done the hard work in getting started, in adding new things and cutting out non-supportive patterns.

Remember "The Voices"...have they taken full hold of your mind yet? Or have you silenced them into submission?

We believe in transparency and being here as supportive, compassionate guides. During the past few days were you tempted at all to eat the foods that you were releasing?

If so please be kind and gentle with yourself, this is part of the process. That statement always turns some heads because so many use shaming as a motivator under the guise of accountability. Let's be real.

If you did get tempted or if you gave into those voices then it helps you to identify and accept that they are real. We can fight an opponent that is real; it's the ones that are made up that are harder to beat.

If you prefer a more compassionate approach to managing your relationship with those voices, please visit our website to listen to Suzanne's audio recording on making friends with your subconscious mind.
http://40DaysToFreedom.com/resources

Your action step for today is to flood your mind and body with a substance that can wash away all of your toxins - WATER!

Drink Twice, Eat third.

Increased appetite is often a sign of dehydration. Unless it has been longer than 3 hours since you've eaten a meal, drink water the first two times you feel hunger pangs.
Hungry after filling your stomach twice with water?

You're actually hungry.

What are you waiting for? Eat something!

Begin increasing your water consumption daily until you consume **1 gallon** of pure water per day.

The specific ratio to calculate your ideal daily water needs is ½ of your body weight (lbs.) of water in oz.

So if you are a 130lbs you would need 65 oz. of water per day.

Note that this calculation is only accurate for a well-hydrated person and considering that the majority of the population is dehydrated we encourage the full gallon.

Empty water.

Most of the water we drink today is polluted or 'empty'. Tap water is heavily contaminated with chlorine, fluoride and even has shown traces of contraceptive pills.

Filtered or distilled water is void of any beneficial minerals because it's all been evaporated or filtered out.

Do you remember learning about osmosis in chemistry class? Minerals move from areas of high concentration to low concentration in what we call the chemical hippie effect... they just wanna be free!

If you're drinking 'empty' water then your body will leach bone, teeth and free minerals out of your cells in order to find a balance. That's not good.

Journal Questions

What do you notice about your appetite when you're drinking enough water (around 1 gallon per day)?

How has your energy changed with the increased water?

What symptoms or pains have you noticed decrease since you've added in more water?

Day 20

We are what we repeatedly do. Excellence therefore is not an act, but a habit.

~ Aristotle

Today we offer one of the most powerful habits that can influence your physical, mental and emotional success/freedom. Often it's the simple things that can have dramatic impact and this action step is an example of that.

Do routine morning cardio, 6 days a week.

This habit of doing a cardio-dominant exercise first thing in the morning, particularly on an empty stomach, will have a huge impact on your body, mind and the connection you feel to your higher self.

"A person's success is largely determined by the rituals they have in their life. ***How we do anything is how we everything****, so therefore just by examining how someone spends their* ***first*** *and* ***last*** *hours of the day is a window into the success they'll achieve now and in the future."*

There are so many layers to this effect that we could write a short book on just those, alone.

Please go to:
http://40DaysToFreedom.com/resources for videos on this routine, its impact and ideas to keep it fresh, including a download of a High Intensity Interval Training (HIIT) program.

Whether you rise and go to the gym, take to the streets outside for a stroll or a jog or you decide to stay indoors for convenience or controlled climate, you can make it very simple, efficient and effective with a few simple guidelines:

1. **Do it first thing when you wake up.**
2. **Do it on an empty stomach**
3. **You can drink water, and if you must, coffee**
    a. **(Keep the coffee black to avoid stomach aches)**
4. **Go continuously for a minimum of 8 minutes**
5. **Observe your thoughts, internal conversation, feelings and mood (before, during and after)**

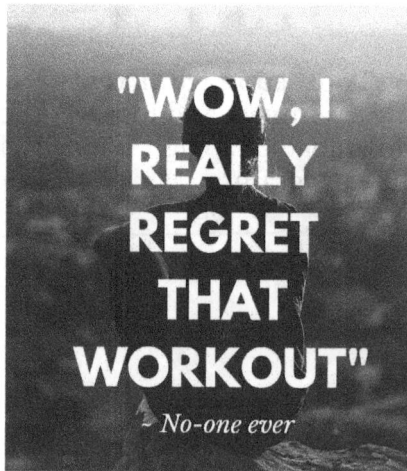

"WOW, I REALLY REGRET THAT WORKOUT"
~ No-one ever

Journal Questions

By now you will have felt the impact of journaling on your mind and routine. Perhaps you have noticed the times when you wanted to skip what is essentially a very short practice (morning cardio).

The times you took action, though, are the times to focus on. The choice to do it even if you didn't feel like it is what builds more character within you, and that is one of the layers that morning routine cardio has on your life - and dare we say - your soul.

How do you feel when you first wake up?

How does your internal conversation change during or after the short workout?

How do you feel after you're done or after having a shower?

How does it impact your energy throughout the day?

Day 19

You will never be free until you free yourself from the prison of your own false thoughts.

~ Philip Arnold

Before you picked up this book we imagine that there were some things you would have thought or said that you could *not* do. Maybe many of them.

Our goal has always been to free you from the prison of your own false thoughts or limitations.

As you've learned, these false thoughts or limits may have been installed by other people or from events that no longer exist in your life.

Today you'll let go of more that doesn't serve you, plan and make decisions that are in line with *your* desired lifestyle, and claim your freedom.

By placing the choice of when to eat certain foods back into *your* hands you can truly have your cake and eat it too - rather than follow other people, societal norms or old habits and appetite patterns which keep you trapped in a cycle that for some, never ends.

Cut your carbs after 3pm.

Eat carbs with the meals you eat before 3pm, where you can eat any gluten-free grains you choose. If you want the occasional pasta dish, fine. Choose quinoa and rice pasta from your local health/grocery store, eat ½ of your meal at noon and then the other half 2.5 hrs. later.

Why?

This will keep your furnace burning and give you more energy that you will be able to burn off during the day.

By removing these starchy foods from the evening, you allow your digestive tract to rest as your body winds down for the day.

You will end up burning stored body fat or "sugar stores" for the remainder of the evening instead of burning more of what you eat.

We have experienced this as having a significantly positive effect on hormones later in the day, when the growth and recovery hormones are rising and stress hormones are decreasing. We have felt these benefits in our own progress and have witnessed them in hundreds of clients making this change.

Look Forward!

After you've completed your 40 Days to Freedom it is okay to have carbs after 3pm *on occasion*.

This is *freedom*!

Remember, we are all different and *you* need to monitor how *you* feel and if you need a little more non-starchy or low-starchy carbs in the evenings. (Use the "**meal tachometer tool**" we have to help you gauge the effectiveness of every meal).

http://40DaysToFreedom.com/resources

Journal Questions

(Use the "meal tachometer tool")

How do you feel when you eat a meal that is primarily made up of fat and protein?
(Better, same, worse)

How do you feel when you eat a meal that is primarily made up of vegetables and protein?
(Better, same, worse)

How do you feel when you eat a meal that is primarily made up of starches and protein?
(Better, same, worse)

Day 18

**Don't stop when it hurts,
pain is temporary.**

**Quitting, however,
lasts forever.**

Today, contemplate your freedom. Freedom from foods you thought you had control over, yet they had control over you.
Freedom to choose, rather than rely on foods and drinks to shift your energy and emotional state.

Freedom from external negative influences that had you making choices and actions that only left you feeling bad, critical and disappointed in yourself.

As the quote on the opposite page says, pain is temporary and as the weeks progress you will find that it gets easier and easier and more part of your way of life.

Your action steps for today are to feed or "pay" your metabolism. We'll tell you how in a moment. First, let's explore some of what you may or may not have experienced this week.

Whether you've been able to completely stay away from soda/sugar & gluten or not is fine. If you haven't, that's okay, you have at least taken steps toward giving it up. A day off is better than no day off.

A breakfast with more protein and no bread is a win.

What's more, it is often a *beneficial* part of the process to eat those foods again when you decide/make the goal to release them.
Why?
Because of the rocks in your belly!

This is how we describe the pain you feel when you start to re-sensitize to gluten and other foods that your digestive tract/gut doesn't like.

We embrace the fact that we sometimes 'slip up', as some may call it.

We don't see it as a slip up if it helps someone to realize and accept that their body *does* perform and feel better without gluten!

This is one of the ways we can successfully re-establish the communication between the brain and gut brain that we mentioned in an earlier chapter. This kind of awareness is what will begin to repair that relationship in your body as you hone your "listening" skills.

Let's get paid!

Now, back to "paying" your metabolism, and our recommendations for how to do that.
Think of your metabolism as your body's engine, like in a car.

It is where the fuel gets burned and therefore it is what drives all of the car's processes to move and run.

Your metabolism can also be thought of as a bank account. The more you deposit into your account the more comfortable it is with allowing you to spend.

Consider if you were to get a paycheck each morning. *Every* morning. How comfortable would you be in spending most or all of your money today?

Now contrast that with how you would feel if you got paid once every three months.

With daily pay, you may get a smaller check each time compared to what you'd get paid per quarter, however the way you'd feel would be more **secure**.

Our bodies operate very similarly to this, and that is why we encourage you to **increase the frequency and amount of meals you eat per day.**

Start by adding in one extra meal or snack. Ideally you want to "pay" your body with food **every 2.5-3 hours**.

Start with your first meal of the day and add 2.5 -3 hours to know when a good *rough* time is for you to eat something again and so on throughout the day. By now you're eating more than just 3 times per day.

Make sure that when you eat again you have some **protein** as part of that meal. The protein will make sure that you stay full longer and will keep your blood sugar stable, thereby decreasing cravings for sugar.

Journal Questions

How do you feel about food?

What has changed? Energy? Mood?

What regrets do you have about quitting something in your past?

Day 17

It's not selfish to do what's right for you.

~ Mark Sutton

Let's Get Serious about Shackles... Let's talk traps.

Traps in this context are things like client dinners, girls' night and other situations where you are encouraged or peer-pressured into behaving (and eating) a certain way.

While this may be the norm, or typical event, the trap only exists in your own mind. *You* decide whether you eat foods you don't want to eat, or aren't in line with what you want.

If you have developed many social reasons for why you're not able to stay on track or why you struggle to find the time to do what's right for you, then it may be an important time to examine how you feel about your worthiness, deservedness and selfishness.

From an early age, we're often made *wrong* for being selfish, yet it's how we come into this world, attempting to survive and get our needs met by those around us.
When did this shift for you? When did *you* decide that looking out for your health - mentally, emotionally and physically - was selfish?

We encourage you to examine this as it may help you to see through a window to your habits and patterns, and your *reasons* when you don't get the results.

Do you need to go out to entertain clients for your work/career? Maybe.
Do you need to eat biscuits and gravy, French toast or pizza? No.

We've worked with clients who are shackled to their persona and felt they needed to eat, drink or act in a way that keeps up with the expectations of their audience. Consider when you go to see your favorite singer in concert and he or she sings and performs in a certain way. You'd expect that, every single performance.

But what if they didn't? What if they reinvented themselves? What if they dared to be different and started a new trend? New clothes? New sound? New style?

Do you think that would ever work?

It *has* worked: Madonna, David Bowie, Prince, Bob Dylan and so many others have done it time and time again.

So we invite you to be different, to "go against the grain" in more ways than giving up that slice of pizza!

Here are our best tips for keeping your freedom while eating out or entertaining clients at dinners:

Eat something before you arrive.
What we call "emergency nut supply" has served our clients for years.

This is a simple trick of keeping some organic, raw nuts (salted is fine) with you in a small zip lock bag, or buying them in snack size bags ready to go.

Before you arrive to the restaurant, make sure that you have at least a handful of nuts. The fat content will reduce your urges for bread when they offer or bring it to the table, and sugar when you start looking at the menu.

Start with lots of water.

As soon as you arrive, start drinking lots of water and refuse the initial offer for an alcoholic drink. This will pre-hydrate you and mobilize your digestive enzymes to be ready when your food comes.

If your clients attempt to coerce you into drinking, especially if they attempt to use the "we're buying" or "we'll be offended" approach, there are a number of ways to handle this.

If you do drink and would like a drink, say that you would "love to have a really nice drink (of your style, i.e. wine or liquor) with your meal and right now you haven't decided what you'll be having.

This will essentially help you to skip on 1-2 drinks compared to your clients.

If you don't drink, then you likely already have your preferred method of dealing with that scenario!

For the main course, focus on your choice of protein (ideally animal protein, however if you are vegan/vegetarian choose your preferred kind) and asking for whatever vegetable(s) appeal most.

Most restaurants will accommodate your request for substitutions, even if you have to ask a few times in a few different ways, and you can typically substitute a high starchy carb such as mashed potatoes or fries for a vegetable dish, grilled or steamed.

Once you get your meal, ask for some REAL butter and load that onto the veggies. You're welcome! (We'll explain the rationale for this more thoroughly in the next chapter).

So you've handled the alcohol and the main course, however maybe it's the desserts that get you.

For dessert, choose fattier things such as crème brûlée, panna cotta or traditional cheesecakes over pastry, pie or anything bread-like.

The fat will slow down the effect of any sugar in the dessert limiting your insulin spike, which will limit further cravings of alcohol or other sugary foods.

It will also limit how quickly that food is shuttled into your fat cells, giving you more time to burn it off.

Journal Questions

Where have you been giving your power up to others?

Contemplate your worthiness. Do you compare it to others?

Are there certain people you would place above you in terms of worthiness? (This would look like you putting others' wants or needs before your own).

Whose permission do you feel you need to be able to make choices that serve *your* best interests?

Day 16

Those who celebrate the small victories and simple pleasures win the game over and over again.

Today we invite you to create a treat schedule for yourself.
In order to create it in alignment with your freedom goals, it is *vital* that you understand our **80/20 Rule**.

Implement the eating habits that we've shared in this book 80% of the time, and more ideally with a customized, genetic-based nutrition program guided by us visit:
http://40DaysToFreedom.com/freedom-to-eat

The other 20% of the time you can have freedom to eat whatever you desire. That said, we invite you to focus that 20% on a single day of the week, and to continue to be conscious of avoiding the more harmful foods for your body.

You may have heard about "cheat days" from other people and essentially those are binge days, where quality and portion-size are typically thrown out of the window and people eat as much as they can of anything not on their typical diets.

While we DO NOT agree with *any* form of binge eating or drinking, we support the idea of what we prefer to call "treat days".

Indulging in treat days builds your self-control muscles and also stimulates a powerful protein that is created inside your fat cells called Leptin. Leptin tells your brain how to set your metabolism. It controls whether you ramp up your fat burning or slow it down, to a halt.

Where we talk about increased meal frequency helping to pay your metabolism, Leptin is connected to fat stores. For survival we are hardwired to slow down our metabolism as our fat stores become depleted. Stored fat, after all, serves as energy reserves in times of famine.

This "Leptin switch" can be manipulated when we consume some healthy fats to provide our body with a sense of safety from famine!

By eating a meal high in fat we trigger the release of Leptin, which had previously dropped due to the body realizing that fat levels, stored or consumed, have been on the decline.

This intermittent treat kickstarts Leptin and thereby kickstarts our metabolism.

When it comes to stress our bodies are influenced heavily by the adrenal glands. These glands release our stress hormones, which are designed to shut down the burning of fat. The more stress we are under the more of those hormones are released and one in particular, Cortisol, is responsible for belly fat accumulation.

What do your adrenals love? Schedule. Consistency.

This is why we often see people with very organized lives in relatively good shape even if they say that they never exercise.

What can you do today to diminish your stress level?

We invite you to create a treat day, which is very much a part of your freedom program.

This would be a consistent day per week where you will allow yourself to have one meal that contains one of the following attributes:

- Whatever you have been craving all week that you seem to struggle doing without. This is helpful because our minds obsess on what we *can't* have. In this case you are allowed to have it, just in limited quantities, so by eating this food/meal your body will feel heard and appreciated.

- A high-protein meal with extra fat. This would be like having the steak with vegetables and adding butter or coconut oil on top of the veggies, as mentioned in the previous chapter.

- High fat meal, lower in protein **and low in carbs.** This may be something like the desserts we mentioned also in the previous chapter - crème brûlée, panna cotta, or cheesecake.

Journal Questions

Contemplate and schedule your treat days. What foods would you choose?

Which day of the week would you schedule to eat them?

What strategies could you come up with to help you be strong through the week so that you stick to your treat schedule?

Day 15

If you don't jump, you'll never fly!

Take the leap and let go!

Today we introduce a highly powerful and transformative process to you. We've needed to wait until this time to reveal it to make sure that those who use it have progressed through the foundation principles and are seriously committed to achieving freedom.

We offer you, Mapping Across!

This technique literally *rewires* your brain and links something desirable with something undesirable, for the purpose of instantly developing distaste for the previously desirable thing. The goal here is to replace shackles with *choice*, especially if you "can't live without it", by forcing you to choose that thing despite a psychological barrier having been placed against it.

Initially you may need to break free from the shackles by developing such repulsion that you don't want the food or drink. We trick the brain to go from trapped to free!
Essentially we take the food you're a slave to, and switch the connection in your brain to one that you dislike or downright hate!

Sound like fun?

Just like after a breakup, where you may need "*space*" from another person before you are truly free following releasing the energy of **attachment**, you may likewise require "space" from this food.

If you have any apprehension or anxiety about breaking up with a food then we offer a very powerful statement that has helped many people get through this very thing for years... ready?

"I'm sorry *(insert food name),* we need to have a little break. It's not you though.... It's me."

Mapping across can be applied to a number of things to transform your behavior and achieve extraordinary results. Today we use it in the context of food and to help you "take the leap" **and let go!**

Journal Questions

What foods are you struggling with omitting from your diet, even if you know it is damaging to your health?

What foods utterly repulse you?

Watch a video example of a Mapping Across and follow the Mapping Across audio to guide you through releasing your attachment to a food/drink.

Go to http://40DaysToFreedom.com/resources

Day 14

If you always put a limit on everything you do, physical or anything else, it will spread into your work and into your life.

There are no limits.

There are only plateaus, and you must not stay there, you must go beyond them.

~ Bruce Lee

Comfort is the epitome of a plateau. It is creating a situation that is stagnant, known and familiar. By that very description it is void of growth, expansion and risk.

To be free of limitations and plateaus in our lives and in our health it is essential for us to keep pushing our comfort zones, stretching them to reach further and just as we have done so, move the target again and repeat.

A saying that we love is ***"If we're not growing, we're dying".*** There is no "comfort" in that zone, because if we're not continuing to grow then we are choosing to get closer and closer to our grave. We are winding down, weakening over time and deteriorating.

Think back to things you've overcome that took a level of discomfort to achieve, for example, learning to walk and learning to ride a bike.
You often fell down or struggled *many* times before you were able to cope, and before you achieved competency at an unconscious level.

Journal Questions

What are 3 things you've been able to achieve that took a high level or persistence and perseverance?

1)

2)

3)

Can you identify an area in your life where you have become too comfortable?

How would you feel, looking back on your life, if you shied away from challenge and lived a plain, boring life?

As a dear friend puts it, *"Would you be happy if you spent your whole life in a flat, grey world?"* - Alison Seveon

Day 13

If it doesn't challenge you, it won't change you!

Today we would like to loop back and gather up all of the small challenges and make sure that you are taking ACTION.

Please, please make this a book that you put into practice and not something that ends up being an entertaining read, or something that simply gets the cog wheels in your mind turning (though that's a valuable change too).

Quite simply we're asking you to cut the crap.

Bad dairy:

Milk from conventionally farmed cows contains high amounts of pus because the cows get mastitis (inflammation of the udder) due to over-milking.

There is actually an allowable limit for pus built into dairy manufacturing laws. The USDA allows up to 750 million pus cells per liter of milk (just over a quart)!

Add to this the fact that these cows are loaded with growth hormones that consequently interfere with *your* hormones.

Substitute all bad dairy with organic, pasture-raised, non-homogenized dairy.

Homogenized milk, by the way, is when milk is spun at very fast rates to burst the fat molecules so that the cream doesn't rise to the top and so that people don't get grossed out by the *natural* process and natural separation of *real* milk. Ha!

Creamers:

These so often have synthetic ingredients, artificial sweeteners and preservatives that cause more harm than if you simply had high quality cream (following the above guidelines). Do you really need this in your coffee though?

Substitute creamer with a ¼ teaspoon of coconut oil or use half & half from grass-fed cows.

Splenda®:

Did you know that Splenda® is **chlorinated** sugar? Need we say more?

Use stevia instead... heck, use *real* sugar instead of chlorinated sugar!

Fruity yogurts

Many people choose fruity yogurts as a way to convince themselves that they are eating a healthy snack, when in fact there are far more sugars than you'd ever consume if you simply added the fruit yourself.

Food manufacturers take almost any chance they get to add sugar to foods because it is such a highly addictive substance. Lab rats actually preferred sugar water to *cocaine* in a recent study!

Substitute these fruited yogurts with plain yogurt and add your own ingredients to flavor.

For a wonderful nut-based, grain-free cereal with yogurt recipe visit **http://40DaysToFreedom.com/resources** and look for "*grain-free cereal alternative*".

High Fructose Corn Syrup

Did you realize that this stuff is *everywhere*?!

Here is just a short list of foods that contain High Fructose Corn Syrup that few people know about:

- Pickles,
- Ketchup or BBQ sauce
- Those same fruity yogurts just mentioned
- Fruit spreads, jam, jelly
- Nut butters
- Certain brands of granola bars or oat bars
- Many popular brand name cereals
- Salad dressings - (store bought or restaurant)

Journal Questions

In our house we encourage our children to taste new foods *before* they speak with an opinion about them. We consider this to be a good preparation for life!

Follow this advice and cut the crap above!

How has this book opened your eyes to the food industry?

Where do you think you were being duped? What were you consuming innocently before, and now choose to avoid?

Day 12

One reason people resist change is because they focus on what they have to give up, instead of what they have to gain.

~ Unknown

Appreciate what you've achieved so that you can attract and create more of it.

Today it is important to look back and see how far you've come. This is no time to judge the journey; we simply need to measure it.

Look at how you felt when you picked up this book. How do you feel now?

Today what have you gained so far on your steps to freedom that you can share with others?

You have gained something that is so important, and perhaps one of the last things you'll think of at this stage...

Insight & Experience.

Take Action and Pay It Forward

Who in your life could benefit from your experience? Who could be moved, motivated or *(fill in the blank)* by hearing about your transformation so far?

This does 2 powerful things:

1. It helps someone else. You take a step forward as a leader. We all have greatness and the power to influence within us and there are people who may only be able to get a breakthrough by hearing *your* story. It could be that they resonate with your background, your pain, your struggle and your situation.

2. It reinforces your success. It highlights the changes you've made and ingrains them at a deeper level. Einstein said that you only really understand something when you can teach it simply, so this act helps them *and* helps you.

Journal Questions

What insight and experience have you gained so far?

What is a key win or breakthrough you've had so far?

What are 3 things that are part of this endeavor that you're grateful for?

1)

2)

3)

Who do you know that you would like to see transform?
(Maybe share a copy of this book for them and share your experience, breakthroughs and successes)

Day 11

Commitment is doing what you said you were going to do, long after the mood you said it in has left you!

Today is clean up day.

This kind of cleaning up is to create congruence from your thoughts to your words to your actions.
Congruence means agreement, compatibility or even togetherness.

Take stock of what you're still doing that you said you'd change at the beginning of this program or at some point throughout it.

Observe what you still have not put into action that you said you would do as part of this program.

As we invite you to clean up any conflicts or contradictions around these areas it is a time for you also to offer forgiveness to anyone who has contributed to this misalignment and also to offer forgiveness for *yourself.*

The past does not equal the future, however doing the same thing over and over certainly won't garner a new result.

Journal Questions

What commitments have you made to other people that you have broken?

What have you not fully committed to that you said you would (even if just to yourself)?

Who has broken agreements or commitments with you in the past?
(How did this make you feel? Have you forgiven them?)

Day 10

Happiness is when what you think, what you say and what you do are in harmony.

~ Mahatma Gandhi

How do you bring harmony to your life and with your relationship to food?

How do you avoid relapse and maintain your success?

We're going to be upfront. Balance is not the aim here, as in life balance is unattainable.

Truly, what would balance look like to you? If you were to "balance the scales" the line would be flat, correct?
Where in life do we achieve a "flat line"?

When our hearts stop and we die.

So the goal is less about balance and more about harmony. Harmony is having all aspects of your body, mind and life in alignment and playing supportive roles with each other.

If you need to put a lot of focus or energy into your physical arena of life, your mental and emotional arenas support with motivation, drive, strategy and focus.

When it is time to emotionally connect with someone, your physical body gives you the stability and presence to express that connection.

It's all about creating a dream team with your conscious mind, your subconscious mind, your physical body and your emotions.

When these "play" together well you will experience a flow and ease in life that most of us strive to attain!

This is our goal for you.

This is the ultimate freedom we wish for you.

The question is, do YOU want it badly enough?

Happiness is when
what you **think**, what you **say**
and what you **do** are in harmony.

- Mahatma Gandhi

Journal Questions

If you were to give yourself a score out of 10 for how much in-harmony your thoughts, words, and deeds are, what would it be?

Where do you feel you are best at being in alignment?
(*Choose from* Thoughts, Words, Deeds)

Where do you feel you need the most improvement to be in alignment?
(*Choose from* Thoughts, Words, Deeds)

Day 9

You are a product of
your environment.
So choose the environment
that will best develop you
toward your objective.

Analyze your life
in terms of environment.
Are the things around you
helping you toward success -
or are they holding you
back?

~ W Clement Stone

Today we focus on removing the "dead weight" to your health and therefore help you elevate your quality of life.

Imagine a hot air balloon.
What keeps it from floating off into the air at any time? They are the sandbags or weights tied to ropes over the edge of the basket.

What lifts it up and drives it is the hot air created by the burner above the opening of the balloon.

What is important to note is that no matter how much hot air you create under the balloon, it is necessary to remove the "dead weight" that is holding it down otherwise it'll never be able to lift off.

This is why releasing negative emotions was so important early on in this book and why you can *continually* release what's negative in your life.

We also need to release disempowering beliefs, as we know they affect what we think we are capable of and the behavior or action we take.

Note that sometimes defeat originates deep in the mind and grows through doubt and the idea of failure. Rid that from your mind.

Use the following questions and the free guided-audio available at
http://40DaysToFreedom.com/resources to release these from your subconscious, then listen to the success audio to reprogram your mind with a new operating system.

**If you can't fly, then run,
if you can't run, then walk,
if you can't walk, then crawl,
but whatever you do,
keep moving forward!**

~ Martin Luther King, Jr.

Journal Questions

What disempowering beliefs have you noticed come up for you?

Where have you been saying that you can't do something?

What have you wanted to do that you have not put action or energy into, yet?

What would you start today if you were guaranteed to succeed?

Day 8

You are never too old to set another goal or to dream a new *dream*

~ C.S. Lewis

You set a goal and it's no longer desirable.
You *can* adjust it!

Ben: *"For years in my clinic many female clients would come to see me and initially say that they didn't want 'Madonna arms'.*

They wanted change, just not too much. They wanted people to notice, just not too much.

It kinda made me realize how often people are imprinted with the idea that their goals/ideas are "too much" early on in their childhoods. What almost always happened, however, was that once they achieved some level of success and started to see a little bicep bump or feel their arm be tighter they would remark about how they wanted more of that!"

One of the reasons for this is that people don't really know how they would feel that far in advance, or around something they don't know about or have experience with. Women who were not in shape saw Madonna's arms as grotesque or extreme, until they saw their own arms get tighter, stronger and sexier. With this experience - a mix of physical feeling and emotional boosting from compliments they received - they now shifted their opinion on what they wanted.

Knowing this phenomenon occurred regularly, it is important to keep this in mind when listening to and working with clients.

Appreciating where they are when they walk in the door and also holding the vision for where they may go in the future is all part of effective and empathetic coaching.

“If I asked people what they wanted, they would have said *a faster horse.*”

~ Henry Ford

Journal Questions

What new ideas, goals and dreams have emerged for you since you started this program?

If you could update or add to your goals, what would you add now?

What did you think you wanted that you now no longer want?

What did you *not* think was possible or did *not* want at the onset of this program that you now think you can or want to achieve?

Day 7

Enter every activity without giving mental recognition to the possibility of defeat.

~ Paul J Meyer

Today is all about awareness.

Awareness is such a powerful step in your own journey and we've used this with such great effect to hide deeper intentions from our conscious mind.

Use today as a very important day to expand your focus in the area of the changes you've made and the changes that have happened around you. In this way **your momentum feeds your motivation.**

Allow us to give you an example with posture.
Awareness is one of the most important and effective strategies when helping someone to retrain and improve their posture.

That said, asking someone to be aware of their own posture is like asking a teenager to clean their room, you can ask all you want and they will ignore you, maybe even more *because* you asked.
Even subconsciously.

Therefore, what we do is ask someone to become acutely aware and critical of *other* people's postures.
This gives the critical part of your mind something to do, and that enrolls it onto your success team.

Now you'll notice the people who stand with one hip sticking out, you'll notice the sloucher in the subway or at their desk. The person whose face is way too close to their computer screen or the person whose head is almost hanging forward off of their neck.

You'll be far more aware of your own posture, because your ego doesn't want to be like those people that you mind was just criticizing.

That is how you enroll your inner critic onto your success team. It will be critical anyway, so why not get it on your side?

Today, become very aware of other people's language.

One specific thing to observe is "**negatives**".

Notice how many times they say these sabotaging words:

Can't - in our opinion the *worst* 4-letter c-word

Try - allowing the possibility for failure
"Do or do not. There is no try." ~ *Yoda*

But - this indicates an "*either/or*" mentality and epitomizes the shackled mindset. It is an expression of being internally split.

Should - referring to, in a word, obligation. Highlighting the emotional cage the person is in. Potentially riddled with guilt or shame and living in its shadow.

Journal Questions

What did you notice about the way people talk about themselves?

What did this help you notice about how you speak about yourself?

What did you notice about how people speak about their obligations?

What did you notice about they way people break/keep their commitments?

How has my lifestyle changed?

Who has changed around me?

- **Friends**

- **Colleagues**

- **Family**

How has the way I think or feel about myself changed?

Day 6

Passion is energy. Feel the power that comes from focusing on what excites you.

~ Oprah Winfrey

Oprah Winfrey was told that she was "too emotional" and "not right for television" early in her career. At this point she could have believed someone else's opinion of her and shrunk to their limitations.

Instead she had faith in her vision and her passion and gave complete commitment to the course, doing whatever she could to make moves in her career.

Over time, her emotional and unique style won the hearts of her audience, the nation and the world, a number of times over.

Where in *your* life could you use more energy through passion and following your heart toward a direction in life where others may doubt you?

Ben: *"For years I pursued a professional basketball career, which at 5'7 was rather unlikely, and I showed up as the underdog in almost every situation. I was often doubted, and always underestimated.*

I was fueled partly by the resistance or the lack of belief from others and mostly from my passion about the game and my role within it. Sometimes what seems to be a negative situation can bring about a strong positive motivator to develop the determination to move toward a goal.

For me the hard work, self-belief and consistent action (often practicing for 6, 7, 8 hours a day to perfect my 3-point jump shot) paid off.

The pinnacle of my career came when I realized my dream, moved to England to play professionally and won Gold in a championship against 22 teams from around the world scoring 36 points -including eight 3-pointers- in the final!"

Journal Questions

Take some time to get clear about what success looks like to you.

Now, go out into your future and place success there.

Please use the audio entitled "**Placing Success in your Future**" for this.

Please be sure to play it when you are sitting or lying down in a relaxed state.
http://40DaysToFreedom.com/resources

Imagine a line that represented the time of your entire existence. Have it pass through your body, so you are in the present and in one direction is the past and in the opposite direction is the future.

If this isn't how you would usually see time, that's ok, just do it for this exercise and then you can put it back where you prefer it.

As you read each word on this page you get more and more relaxed, each letter making your eyes heavier and heavier, your breathing, slower and slower and your whole body feels really, really relaxed, now.

That's right.

You're so relaxed that it seems that you **are**, getting lighter and lighter and you can feel the energy around you **lifting** and pulling **up** to the sky. Any and all noise around you is rushing in through your ears as if it was a loud wind as you **float** higher into the sky.

Your eyes are blinking more frequently and slowly as, you struggle to keep them open, while still reading this.

That's right, you're doing it so well...

Close your eyes for a few seconds and float up above your body... just to prove to yourself that you can do it... then come back and read on...

Now that you are floating look down and see yourself to know that you are floating high above yourself.

As you look in the direction of the future you feel yourself float forward into your future above your timeline.

Float faster out into the future, to a point 20-30 minutes *after* you've successfully completed your goal. Turn around and look back toward the present moment...

Now look down and see your future self, as if you're looking at someone else, and watch as you are celebrating success...

What do you see? What do you hear? What do you feel, now that you've successfully met your goal, and exceeded your wildest expectations?

Now, float back toward now, only as fast as you can observe all of the milestones, signs and achievements along the way that lead you to success.

Look out for images you see that will let you know later that you are on the path to success...

Listen for sounds that you will hear later that let you know that you're on the path to success...

Feel the feelings of confidence and assuredness that you are on the path to success no matter what shows up on the path.

That was *huge*, wasn't it?

Breathe...

Day 5

**Look at life through
the windshield,
not the rear-view mirror.**

~ Byrd Baggett

Today we're focusing on *movement* and *direction*.

Do an activity or workout today that you've never done before.

Learn or play a different sport.

Take a new route for a hike.

Take a lesson in something that will expand your horizons mentally and physically, as this is what inspires your imagination.

As for direction, we are all about moving forward.

Almost every human being, even if they *have* lived in a cave most of their life has had Significant Emotional Events that cause "baggage". Why dwell on those?

We have shown you a powerful Mental & Emotional Release® process and how to put success in your future, yet these are relatively passive ways to create change.

Today take a highly *active* one, for it will energize every cell of your body and serve as a catalyst for change.

We welcome you to download Ben's motivational music track where he integrates high-energy motivational speeches with euphoric music.

Download the mp3 at:
http://40DaysToFreedom.com/resources

While listening visualize about the life you have always wanted.

Imagine the person you've always wanted to be.

Dream of the things you've always wanted to do.

Feel the experiences you've always wanted to have.

"Go confidently in the direction of your dreams! Live the life you've always imagined!"

- Henry David Thoreau

Journal Questions

Did you know that the way memories and dreams activate our brains are essentially the same?
Therefore, what would you dream about being ahead of you rather than recollecting what's behind you?

What memories could you let go of to help you move forward in life?

What is one thing you need to know to move forward in your life?

Take 5-10 minutes, or as much time as you prefer, to dream about that now. Close your eyes and start to imagine the information coming to you. If you need a visual, look up the way that people can "upload" skills in the movie, *The Matrix*.

Day 4

Many of life's failures are people who did not realize how close they were to success when they gave up.

~ Thomas Edison

Have you heard of the term '3 feet from gold'?

It is a parable about how close someone was to striking gold during the gold rush days.

People would dig and dig for days and when they finally lost hope someone would swoop in and pick up where they left off, only to find that they had quit just 3 feet from gold (illustrated here with diamonds per Suzanne's request)!

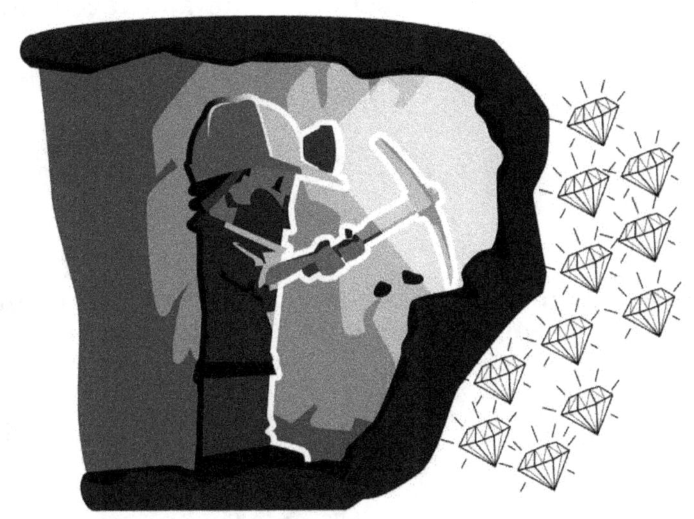

Journal Questions

Where have you given up in the past so close to completing something and regretted it?

When have you persevered and completed something you committed to or really wanted to achieve and felt satisfaction, pride and the feeling that all of the work and dedication was worth it?

Write about how these 2 feelings and situations differ, and which you would like to define you and your character most?

Day 3

If you're tired of starting over, stop giving up!

This book represents your freedom. Whether you've had it before and lost it, or if you feel as though you never had freedom in the areas of food, body image and control.

Freedom is a life choice. A lifestyle.
A **journey**, not a *destination*.

If we were to ask you if you wanted to be free for a day, and you could experience all of the highs and joys of that freedom and then just as soon as you'd experienced it that freedom would be taken away from you, we wonder how you would feel.

Consider then, that this is what happens when people diet cycle. There is a focus on achieving a destination. A strong will and desire to get to that end goal, that taste of freedom, that it appeals more than the sweetest foods or the most fun environments.

What happens when it is achieved?

The desire weakens, the drive loses steam and the yearning for that taste is satisfied. At this point changing the approach that brought us success would be like walking back to a prison or a cage a day or two after being set free!

"There is a complacency that sets in when people feel as though they are on course for success... Most people slow down before the finish line.

We encourage you to speed up!"

- Ben Patwa

We share this simple analogy as an example to inspire people to run powerfully and passionately toward their goal and *speed up* through the finish line!

In a college track meet a runner for the University of Oregon was so far in advance and had the race in the bag, however he started to wave to the crowd to cheer for his performance and slowed down on his way to the finish line.

With a seemingly insurmountable distance to catch up, the runner for University of Washington sprinted with everything he had and lunged for the line to take 1st place and teach a valuable and painful lesson to the complacent runner from Oregon.

(Watch the video of people celebrating too early at **http://40DaysToFreedom.com/resources**).

Journal Questions

When have you stopped taking positive actions after achieving a goal or hitting a milestone, only to fall off of the pedestal and lose the achievement?

When have you felt complacent about results that you've achieved?

What thoughts, distractions or obstacles *repeatedly* show up for you to sabotage you from finishing?

Day 2

Embrace your new I.D.

Embrace your new I.D.

It takes courage, bravery and faith to complete a journey to retrain your mind, release negative emotions and choose new supportive beliefs.

The prize?

You now have a new Identity.

In order to maintain this new identity it is important to create a framework around it. This framework is essentially a new operations manual for your new Identity, your new being.

When working with people who wish to stop smoking, they go through a transformation from someone who smokes to someone who doesn't.

That is ***behavior***.

Remember that behavior is low on the neurological levels, with values, beliefs and identity above it.

What really happens that makes the difference is the change in ***identity***.

The person goes from being a smoker to a nonsmoker.

Journal Questions

Who have you *become* that you weren't, before reading this book?

Who are you now *not,* after reading this book?

What is now possible for you that you didn't think was possible before?

Day 1

**Mastering others is strength.
Mastering yourself is
true power.**

~ Lau Tsu

It's the final day on your countdown to FREEDOM!

Throughout these past 40 days we've been re-wiring you from all directions.

Therefore, it is without a doubt that your values will have shifted because your Identity (who you think you are) has changed.

True power is self-mastery and the path to self-mastery is self-awareness and self-control.

Over the past 40 days you've developed and exercised *both* of these disciplines and it's time to reflect and evaluate your journey.

As you released negative or non-supporting beliefs, it will have affected your values from the top down.

Through controlling and adjusting your environment you made changes to your behavior and certainly your skills/capabilities will have affected your values from the bottom up.

Identity
Beliefs
→ **Values** ←
Capabilities
Behavior
Environment

Please go back to Day 39 and use the Human Values table to elicit your values.

It is important to now examine how those have shifted and be aware of how to live in alignment with them day to day.

We encourage you to come back to this book periodically and use it as a tool to help you re-evaluate how you're living, what's important to you and as a gauge for your environment and how you are orchestrating your life.

Journal Questions

What is important to me in life?

What is important to me in the area of health & wellness?

How do I feel different as a person? How has my identity changed? (What you would say with "I am..." statements)

Freedom Day

Hooray! It's FREEDOM DAY!
.... now what's next?

Just like when you passed your driver's test, the journey is about to begin, rather than being over.

Where will you go?

What will you do?

Who will you be, with the new freedom you have created for yourself?

What is now possible for you, not just in health or fitness, but in every aspect of your life?

Key Wins, Insights & Breakthroughs

What Did You Get From This Book?

We've found that by journaling your response to these questions for 10 minutes per day for 7 days after completing you will retain up to 80% more of the knowledge you've garnered.

Go....

Key Wins, Insights & Breakthroughs

There's no use rowing harder, in the wrong direction.

~ Chinese proverb

It would be wonderful if we could say that your life would be a simple straight line from here forth, and that would be a lie.

Achieving the harmony we've talked about within your lifestyle is a never-ending, winding process.

We are here to help, and we believe that it is our purpose to guide and support you to achieving the most complete, fulfilled and vital life you can.

If you want to learn more about *your* specific genetic requirements for protein, fat, carbohydrate and how your dominant hormonal systems influence more about when and where you store body fat, we have created a program called **Freedom To Eat™**.

Customized Nutrition Program
Freedom to Eat™

Within this program you receive the Advanced Level Metabolic Typing test to identify your dominant system for creating energy from food.

You will also receive an analysis of your dominant hormonal system for storing body fat and your individual dominance for alkaline:acidic balance.

All of the popularity over being in an alkaline state has driven people to classify certain foods as acidic vs. alkaline, when in fact foods react differently in different bodies.

Success

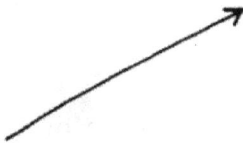

what people think it looks like

Success

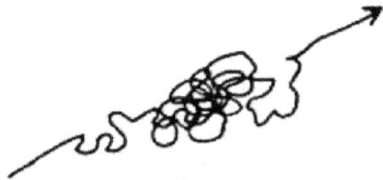

what it actually looks like

We all get there differently. Just like with our Success GPS.

Metabolic Typing® determines 2 very important factors:

#1. Which branch of your autonomic nervous system is more dominant than the other?
Your *sympathetic nervous* system is a 'fight or flight' nervous system, which helps you burn energy, and your *parasympathetic* is a 'rest and digest' nervous system that helps you conserve energy.

The autonomic nervous system takes care of all processes in the body that happen naturally, like your heart rate and breathing. With this basic information you can see how important this is to digesting food and utilizing energy stores in your body.

#2. How fast, or how slow, do your cells convert food into energy?
This is referred to as cellular oxidation and determines if you are a fast or slow oxidizer.

Oxidation is basically how fast or slow the food you eat is turned into energy or stored as fat! If you are 'fast' then that means you convert food into energy quickly.

Again you can imagine how this little piece of the metabolic puzzle will greatly impact your health and weight loss goals!

TIPS: People who are fast oxidizers need to eat heavier proteins and fats because they burn through food faster. If you are a slow oxidizer and turn your food into energy slowly then you should be eating more carbohydrates in your diet!

Once you take a metabolic typing test, it will determine 'your type'.

Protein type: You oxidize food quickly or are parasympathetic dominant. You are hungry often and may crave fat or salt. You may feel lethargic or on edge some days and be a bit of a procrastinator.

Carbohydrate type: You oxidize food slowly or are sympathetic dominant. You don't usually eat much, feel fuller longer and have problems with weight management. You find that you are dependent on caffeine and may have an aggressive, impatient personality and like to work out and achieve goals!

Mixed type: You are neither fast nor slow, parasympathetic or sympathetic dominant. You don't really have cravings for specific food and you don't have issues with weight control. You may be fatigued or nervous often.

"One man's food is another man's poison."
- Hippocrates

Freedom To Eat
Case Studies

"I was struggling with how I looked and felt. I was desperate to lose weight. I was eating what I thought was healthy and visiting the gym regularly but wasn't getting results.
I was tested to see what my Metabolic Type was and I soon discovered I was eating all the wrong foods for ME.

My goal was to feel happy and comfortable in my bikini on my holiday.
It worked! It was amazing!

In 16 weeks I dropped 4 dress sizes, my energy levels improved dramatically and I felt amazing. This is a way of life, no quick fixes, it's not a diet, it's a lifestyle.

Once you understand how it works it's incredibly easy to maintain."

~ Elizabeth W.

"I'd been struggling for the last few years to figure out how to balance exercise and diet and in 5 weeks with just the nutrition coaching I've lost just over 9lbs and it's been fabulous!

My body's gone through a lot of changes, I'm seeing my abs again for the first time in years!"

~ Stephanie S.

"What's amazing is that in 6 months I lost a whopping 33.5 inches and 8.6% body fat! It's completely unreal!

Thank you very much!"

~ Dipika K.

If you're not assessing, you're guessing!

We offer comprehensive lab testing to help you achieve optimal health & performance.

More information follows.

The Hormone Map™

Overcome Hormone Imbalance to Drop the Fat, Clear the Fog and Beat Fatigue At Any Age

This is the most comprehensive, drug-free program to balance hormones naturally. Created by a Certified Functional Diagnostic Nutritionist and a Registered Nurse.

Are you suffering *any* of these 3 signs of Hormone Imbalance?

Hard to Burn Fat

Are you struggling to burn fat, especially around your belly?

Are you finding that the tricks that you once used just aren't working anymore?

Not Healing or Growing

If your body isn't recovering from exercise, strenuous activities, late nights or you are burned out from striving in your business or career, then Hormone Imbalance may be what's holding you back.

You're up, but not yet awake!

Do you wake up feeling rested, or do you need more sleep, no matter how early you go to bed? Are you energized when you get up in the morning or do you only feel as though you "get going" several hours later?

What's included:
Comprehensive Saliva Lab test:
7 Primary hormones
Cortisol 4 x day
DHEA
Estradiol & Estriol
Testosterone
Progesterone
Melatonin
Tested in a federally certified Laboratory
We pay your lab fees & Express domestic shipping!

Private Members Area - with instructional videos to show you how to balance your hormones drug-free.

Integrated Success Guidebook - Helps you stay accountable on your path through the program.

Your Hormone Map™ - A Personalized Protocol designed specifically for you, to bring balance and vitality back into your life safely and effectively.

1hr Private Phone/Skype Consultation - Ask us anything you want, get clarity and gain confidence by knowing What to do, Why to do it & How it'll benefit you.

Weekly check ins - with your Health Coaches/authors Ben & Suzanne.

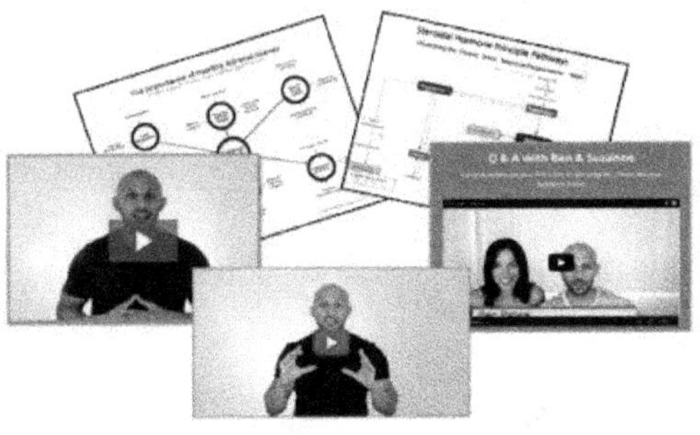

Client Results on The Hormone Map

"I started working with Ben and Suzanne after suffering a rather extreme case of adrenal fatigue while tackling a graduate program and working full time.

I felt so horrible I was inclined to go towards more extreme measures.

After a long review of my situation, Ben and Suzanne recommended trying a more balanced approach.

They gave me supplement recommendations that were far more affordable than most and within two to three days of taking them, I was already feeling better.

Fortunately Ben & Suzanne have a very holistic view of health and can make easy and affordable tweaks that help me regain balance and either feel a lot better or perform a lot better."

~ Ravi C.

"It was a pleasure working with Ben and Suzanne. I'm so happy with the results I've received and everything that I've learned to maintain my good health.

I can't begin to explain in words how wonderful it's been to work through these issues and feel like myself again when I had so much despair before."

~ Carrie C.

"I was having some issues with lack of energy and a general feeling of malaise throughout the day. I was relying heavily on caffeine and other stimulants to power me through my weightlifting and running sessions.

I was referred to Ben and Suzanne to help me look for the underlying cause of my problems.

They "held my hand" as they broke all the scientific jargon down into layman's terms so that I could see just what was going on.

I followed their plan, took the recommended supplements and started to get back to normal energy levels within a few weeks!

I would highly recommend trusting in the advice of Ben and Suzanne to anyone who is looking to feel better, get stronger, more fit and stabilize their energy levels as well as increase their sense of well-being."

~ Mike R.

Food sensitivities test - MRT®

Which of Your Foods are Making You Sick?

We use the most advanced test for identifying all levels of food sensitivities.

Many of the common ailments that you may be suffering from can be linked to hidden food sensitivities.

Headaches, weight gain, skin problems, stomach and digestive issues as well as a myriad of other ailments are often caused by your individual food sensitivities that unless specifically tested for, never get discovered.

On the next page find a test result from Jane's Food Sensitivity Test. Jane eats well, and exercises at a gym once or twice a week. She suffers from migraine headaches and various digestive issues.

After taking this simple test she is now aware of the foods that she has sensitivities to.

Jane is quite surprised to find out that she reacts to bananas and tuna! She often opts for tuna on a salad for lunch since it has long been considered a "healthy" alternative to burgers or sandwiches.

From this brief example, you can see that even more important than eating healthily, you must know what foods are right for YOU!

Everyone has their own hidden food sensitivities.
It becomes obvious if you have a severe allergy to a food, but what if your symptoms are a bit more subtle, albeit persistent?

We believe that everyone should have this test done as soon as possible. Following the recommendations will completely transform your life.

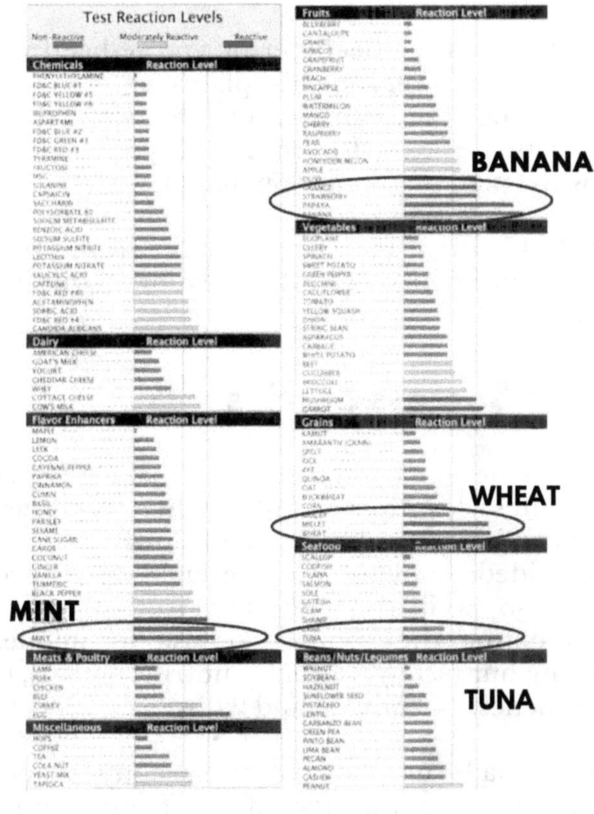

---

*"Jane is quite surprised to find out that she reacts to **bananas** and **tuna**!"*

---

40 Days to Freedom™ **Fitness Program**

A complete program working on your mental *and* physical fitness! The results won't just show on the outside, you will feel them on the inside and they will permeate everywhere in your life - relationships, career, thoughts, attitude & self-image.

Whether you are a beginner or you've been working out for a while, everyone hits plateaus.
We've done the hard work choosing the right combination of exercises so that all you need to do is follow the plan that we give you.

In just 40 days you can benefit from increased energy, confidence and feel happier within your body!

Fitness Success Stories

Quinci came to us determined to make a big change to her lifestyle. After a shift in her living and job situations the excess pounds had slowly crept on and she decided enough was enough! The program worked so well she repeated it 2 times. After implementing the simple exercise techniques and following our tasty yet healthy nutrition plans, Quinci lost 26inches, 7% body fat and 22lbs!

Suzanne had run the gamut of body shapes and fitness levels by the age of 40...from competitive athlete to significantly overweight mother of two, from weight loss, lean limbs and loose skin to a fuller, muscular physique from weightlifting, she was seeking her next fitness challenge. After completing the 40 Days to Freedom Fitness Program, Suzanne kickstarted the momentum toward competing -

coming in 2nd place - in an international Fitness Model Competition just 6 weeks later. *"No matter your fitness goals, this program will provide the education and disciplined approach needed to get results, fast."*

~ Suzanne C.

I had been feeling down on myself because I had put on 15 pounds and had lost the motivation to work out.

When I found this program, I was very excited to get started because I knew it was something I could stick to.
It's very tough to say which part was my favorite because the entire program was enjoyable.

For starters I found the website to be very easy to navigate. It was very organized! Ben and Suzanne did an amazing job of creating recipes, shopping lists and downloadable nutrition guidelines.

The recipes are easy to follow and most important very tasty...at no point on this journey did I feel deprived of anything!

I loved the workout routines because I was able to print out the daily exercises and review the videos before hitting the gym. While at the gym I would often view the videos again before I did the exercise to make sure I had the right form.

I believe that the most beneficial part to me was the support from the private Facebook page. Other participants as well as Ben and Suzanne gave encouragement, suggestions, and support. They were always there to answer any questions I had.

Throughout the 30 days I lost a total of 15 pounds and I have never felt so great! My allergies went away, I find myself sleeping better, and my energy is through the roof."

~ Adriana S.

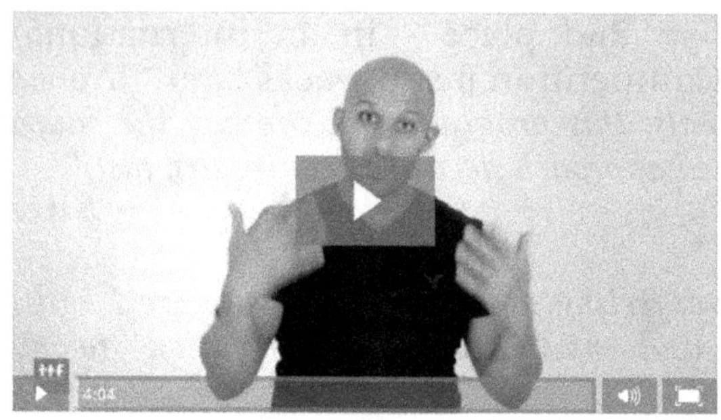

No longer will you worry if you are doing the right things and then end up falling short of your goals. We set you up with everything you need to embark on your transformation. All you need to do is follow the steps for 40 days.

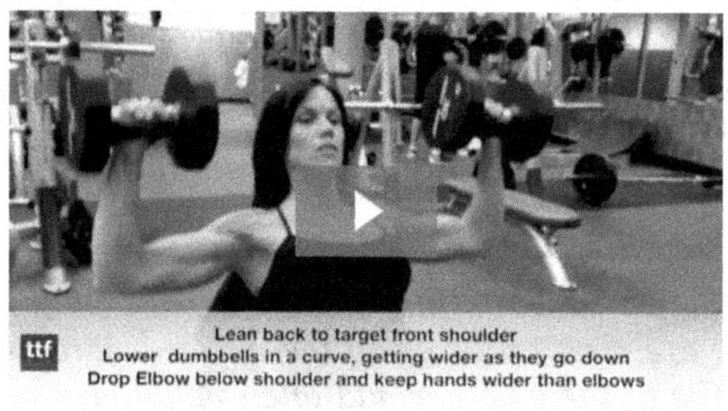
ttf
Lean back to target front shoulder
Lower dumbbells in a curve, getting wider as they go down
Drop Elbow below shoulder and keep hands wider than elbows

Most people don't get their desired results because they don't know what to do, or they don't do the exercises properly. With this program you're never alone, we're *there with you* each workout with instructions and a walkthrough video on your smartphone so that you know what to do and how to do it.

It's like we're your personal trainers in your pocket!

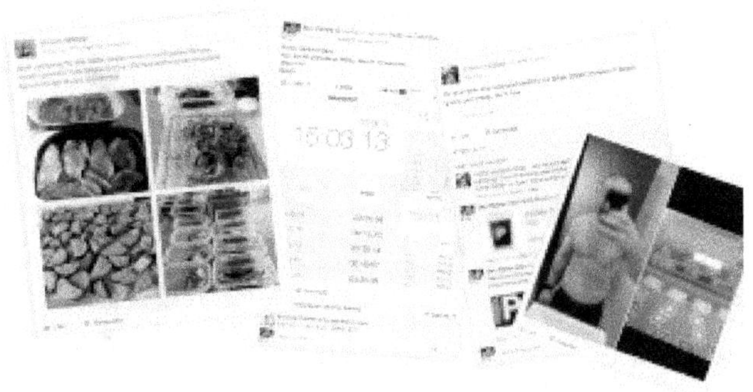

One of the biggest obstacles to success is an unsupportive environment of negative people and situations. We help you solve that with our secure online community forum.

We created a place for you to go to for support and to connect and share with each other anytime you need it, with like-minded people committed to a similar goal of Freedom in 40 days!

Accessible anytime, from any device or on the web, you will have the support you need to help you breakthrough your barriers and take the steps necessary to achieve freedom. Trust us, trust the process and trust yourself.

"The universe doesn't give you what you ask for with your thoughts - it gives you what you demand with your actions."

~ Steve Maraboli

---

40 Days to Freedom

Action Steps, Condensed

30. Public Declaration of Independence
29. Start Your Freedom Journal
28. Increase protein at breakfast & add Freedom Formula supplements
27. Time & Energy Drains
26. Release Draining Foods
25. Coping with Cravings
24. Avoid/limit unsupportive people and environments
23. Place a $/hr on your Health
22. We are what we absorb - add Digestive Enzymes & some high quality fats
21. Drink 1 gallon of pure water per day
20. Do 8+ minutes of morning cardio 6 days/wk.
19. Cut your carbs after 3pm (generally)
18. Pay your metabolism - eat every 2.5-3hrs
17. Shed the shackles when eating out
16. Create a treat schedule - 1 consistent day/wk.
15. Mapping Across
14. Stretch Your Comfort Zone
13. Cut The Crap
12. Pay forward your Insight & Experience
11. Get congruent & complete. Forgive yourself.
10. Happiness is Harmony
9. Remove the "dead weight"
8. Re-evaluate your goal
7. Become aware of your language & thoughts
6. Place success in your future
5. Charge Ahead
4. 3 feet from gold
3. Speed up toward the finish line!
2. Embrace your new I.D.
1. Re-evaluate your values

FREEDOM!

- Notes -

- Notes -

Gratitude & Appreciation

We are so thankful for all of the people who have had an influence on us over the years.

This book is dedicated to our teachers, mentors, colleagues, clients, patients, friends and family who have been part of our journey.

It took a lot of focused energy to write and share this book with you and we are deeply grateful for our strong family unit for the love, energy and support to make this happen.

Many long days into nights and sacrifices were made to be able to dedicate ourselves to creating an original book that will transform its readers.

Special thanks to our children Vivian and Dash who so gracefully endured the process and offered "inspiration kisses" and supreme independence during our most trying moments!

We are grateful for our parents and siblings and for the way we were raised, appreciating organic, whole foods before they were generally valued and the strong work and social ethics instilled in those early years.

Special thanks to Coach Doe Williams, Mrs. Betty Bridge, Clare Condon and all of those who've supported us in becoming the people we are today.

Thanks also to Dan for his brotherhood, Kirsten for her creative input & Jay for his unwavering positivity and enthusiastic support!

It has been a long-held goal of ours to create a paradigm shift in the way that the world views and approaches health.

Our mission is to empower adults as well as children to find *their* unique definitions of freedom, to live by their own guidelines and to follow their path despite any negative influence from the media, society or people around them.

To all of you who crossed our paths, thank you. We are connected, and therefore you are a part of our great legacy.

~ **Ben & Suzanne**

About The Authors

For a collective 30+ years, Ben Patwa and Suzanne Catherine have helped others transform their lives through the practices of Nursing, Functional Diagnostic Nutrition, Physiotherapy/Corrective Exercise Therapy, NLP, Hypnotherapy, Mental and Emotional Release® Therapy, Behavioral Change Therapy and Metabolic Typing®.

Suzanne has two decades of nursing experience in Intensive Care Units at some of the top-ranked hospitals in North America.

Troubled by the common diagnoses she saw in so many patients - Coronary Artery Disease, Stroke, Obesity, Diabetes Type 2 - and learning that so many of them are preventable with education, availability of resources, a shift in lifestyle and the desire to live well, she transitioned into private nursing to have a greater impact on her patients through holistic education and healing.

She has personally run the gamut of physical shapes and sizes, from athletic to anorexic to significantly overweight...to successful competitive fitness model.

She has successfully used the guidelines described in this book to navigate the process to freedom that so many of our readers are desperate to achieve.

She often says, *"Once I knew better, I couldn't forget. This knowledge changed the way I think about food and exercise, and most important, the way I view myself. I simply could not go back to being the person I used to be."*

Ben has been committed to excellence and perseverance from a young age, after growing up as the underdog pursuing a career in Basketball. At 5'7" he was repeatedly told that his dream was impossible and that he should set his sights elsewhere.

Driven by the mindset he shares in this book, he went on to play professionally and scored 36 points, hitting eight 3-pointers, in the championship final to win Gold, defeating 22 countries from around the world.

He became a lifetime student of holistic therapies following his near-death experience when he suffered multiple organ failure at the young age of eighteen.

His resulting resolve to uncover how his body works and his commitment to helping others has fueled his passion for excellence in his field.

Ben successfully built a holistic practice and expert reputation both in his privately owned London clinic and now with clients spanning the globe.

He is popularly known as *"The guy you go to when nothing else has worked".*

Please share how this book impacted you with friends, family and on social media and help us spread our work around the globe!

If you would like Ben & Suzanne to speak or share this information with your staff, school or group please contact us at **support@benpatwa.com** for more information.

www.ingramcontent.com/pod-product-compliance
Lightning Source LLC
Chambersburg PA
CBHW070801280326
41934CB00012B/3004

* 9 7 8 0 6 9 2 6 9 2 8 3 7 *